TATTOO ROAD TRIP—
SOUTHERN CALIFORNIA

BOB BAXTER

PHOTOS BY THE AUTHOR

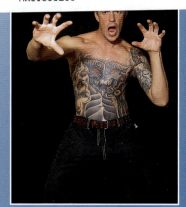

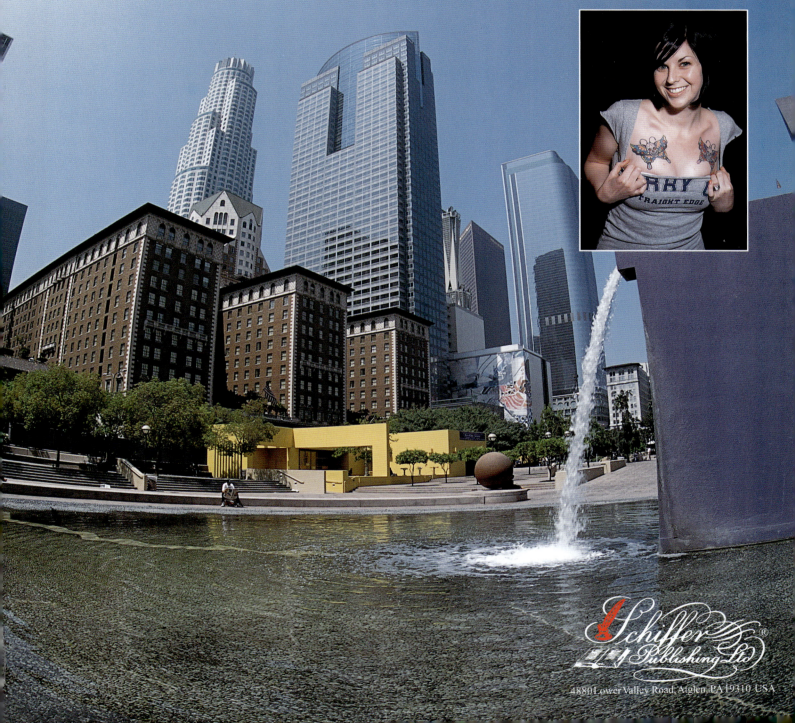

Schiffer Publishing Ltd

4880 Lower Valley Road, Atglen, PA 19310 USA

DEDICATION

For my dear Suzanne

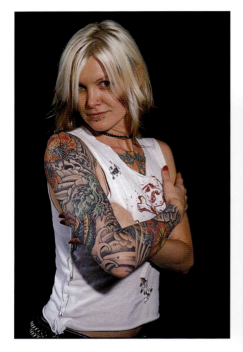
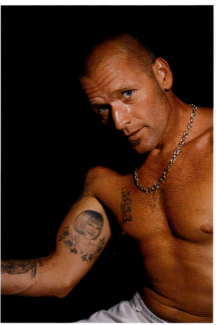
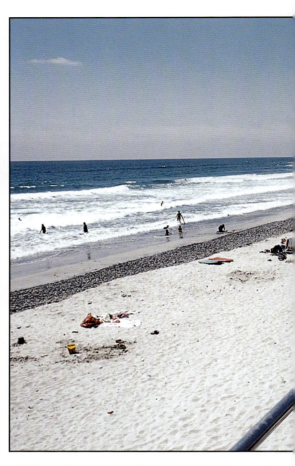

Historical photos courtesy of Tattoo Archive, Berkeley, California.
Cover model, Ann Snair. Tattoos by Riley Baxter
Additional illustration by Theo Mindell.

Designed by John P. Cheek
Cover design by Bruce Waters
Type set in Busorama Md BT/Korinna BT

ISBN: 0-7643-1839-X
Printed in China

Published by Schiffer Publishing Ltd.
4880 Lower Valley Road
Atglen, PA 19310
Phone: (610) 593-1777; Fax: (610) 593-2002
E-mail: Info@schifferbooks.com
Please visit our web site catalog at
www.schifferbooks.com
We are always looking for people to write books on new and related subjects. If you have an idea for a book please contact us at the above address.

This book may be purchased from the publisher.
Include $3.95 for shipping.
Please try your bookstore first.
You may write for a free catalog.

In Europe, Schiffer books are distributed by
Bushwood Books
6 Marksbury Ave.
Kew Gardens
Surrey TW9 4JF England
Phone: 44 (0) 20 8392-8585; Fax: 44 (0) 20 8392-9876
E-mail: Bushwd@aol.com
Free postage in the U.K., Europe; air mail at cost.

CONTENTS

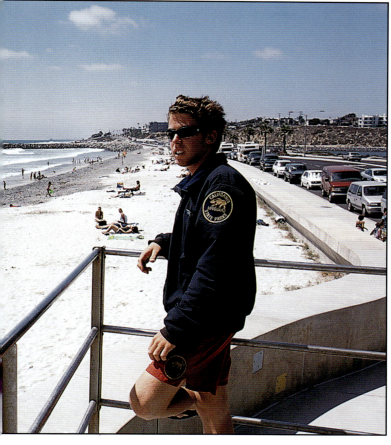

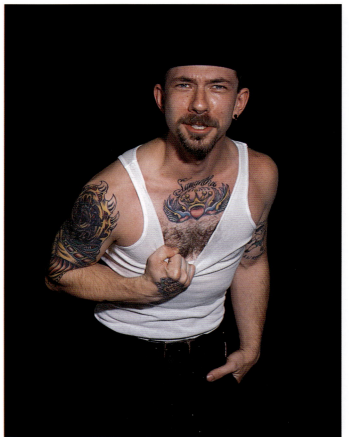

INTRODUCTION

WELCOME TO SOUTHERN CALIFORNIA!

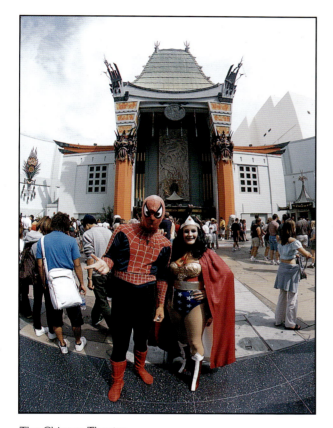

The Chinese Theatre.

It may seem the only planning I do for a *Road Trip* book is select the artists and jot their names on a calendar. Actually, the process involves weeks of research, a bushel basket of personal experience, and endless soul searching. To date, there are approximately 589 tattoo shops in California. Probably two-thirds of those are in the southern part of the state. With an average of 5.3 ink sinkers per shop (just a guess), that adds up to about 2,060 artists to choose from. I whittled that down to 37. And it wasn't easy.

Joe Vegas once told me, "Just make a list, any kind of list, and everyone will want to be on it." Well, I made a list, and, for one reason or another, lots of excellent artists aren't on it. In order to arrive at a manageable number of quality tattooists, someone's going to be left out. A couple I couldn't track down, one was caring for his ill parents, and another's shop was three feet deep in sawdust. I feel badly but I had to move on. For the most part, I selected men and women I'm familiar with, artists with solid reputations or, quite simply, friends I

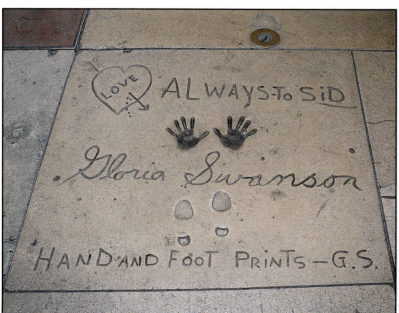

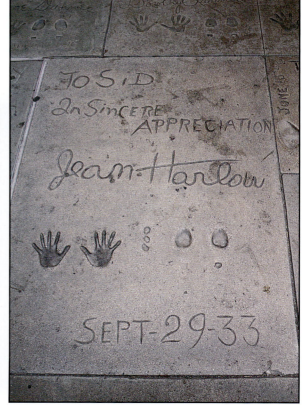

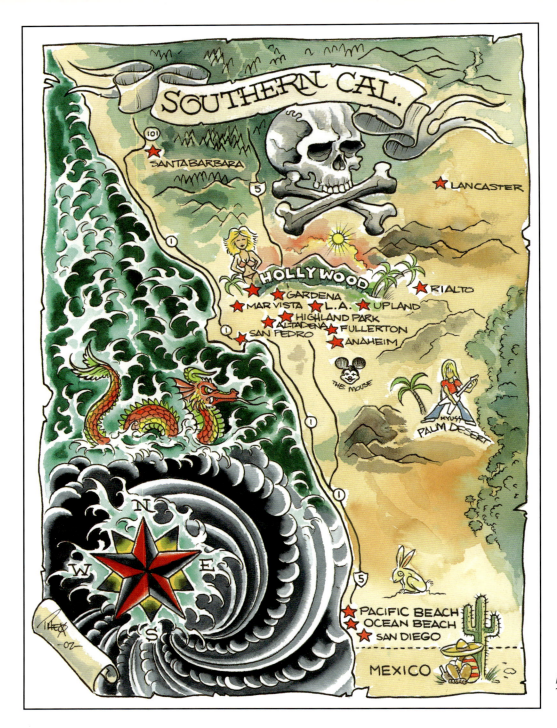

have made during the last six years as Editor in Chief of SKIN & INK Magazine. As my dear, departed father, Pawnee, might say, "I'd be proud to share a hot meal with anyone in this book."

Today, in the early years of the 21st century, tattooing is both more popular and more accepted than ever before. Where once the sight of a tattooed biceps made women faint, children cry, and strong men cower, now it's no big deal. Everyone is on the bandwagon. Everyone loves tattoos.

Bob Roberts of Spotlight Tattoo told me that twice a year he lights up his Harley and rides alone to the Midwest for biker events. "Ten years ago," says Bob, "whenever I'd stop at a roadside diner for a bite to eat, I'd take off the jacket, bare my arms, and, in seven minutes flat, I'd be surrounded by cops. Nowadays, I stop at the very same places, the waitresses run over to my table, pull up their skirts and show me their tattooed butts. Times have changed."

This book is a document, a slice of time in the tattoo history of Southern California. Spread out over 12 weeks, I kept a visual diary of my visits from Santa Barbara to San Diego, from the Pacific Coast to the Inland Empire. Southern California is my home. So, welcome to my neighborhood. Sit back, roll down the window and relax. These are my stomping grounds, the weather's great, and I know lotsa cool places to eat.

—Bob Baxter

DAVE GIBSON
LUCKY'S TATTOO, SAN DIEGO

Rats! It would have been sooooo easy to start with an artist in Pasadena, but no. Pasadena's where I live, but, because of a glitch, I'm off to the home of America's largest military installation, San Diego. Dave Gibson's well-established shop, Lucky's Tattoo, might close, and Dave wanted me to drop by before the classic décor was taken down. That's why I'm a week ahead of schedule.

It's two hours and 15 minutes from my porch to the door of Lucky's. A bit of a haul, but, once the morning fog cleared, the sky turned blue and the clouds came out to play, my heart starting beating in anticipation of interviewing Mr. Dave Gibson. Sure, I spied Dave a couple of times at conventions, but we'd never really talked. I guess I was waiting for the perfect moment to connect up with this famous old-school artist.

The best plan would be to visit all the San Diego shops in one weekend. But Dave put the kibosh on that. He lost his lease after 11 years and might have to move to another location before my June starting date rolled around.

"It's a great shop," he told me. "I really have it where I want it. I'd love for you to take some photos before I relocate."

So much for careful planning. I guess I could report the story out of order. But that wouldn't reflect the true *Road Trip* spirit. So, for integrity's sake, I opted to report the events as they unfold.

WELCOME TO SAN DIEGO

Nixing the convoluted directions supplied on the Internet, Dave told me to take the 5 freeway south to Tenth Street, go to Broadway and then right on Sev-

enth. It worked like a charm. A big hunk of the fun on these road trips is getting there. True, the 5 freeway, the Golden State, is a fairly unimaginative stretch of concrete that extends from Chula Vista on the south to Vancouver, B.C., on the north, but if you want to get somewhere fast, the 5 peels hours off the drive. To me, the only visual excitement was pulling over to the shoulder and photographing a church.

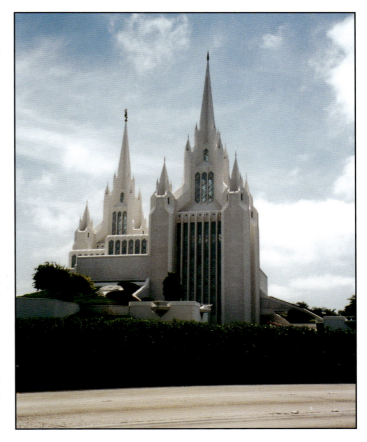

When I turned the corner on Seventh—two hours and 15 minutes on the dot—the shop was on the left. In front of the door was an empty spot. As a bonus, it was Memorial Day Sunday, and parking didn't cost a dime.

Once inside, three young artists, Luke Wessman, Dan Pryor, and Vinnie Almanza, helped me stow my gear. The first thing I noticed was the pedal steel guitar.

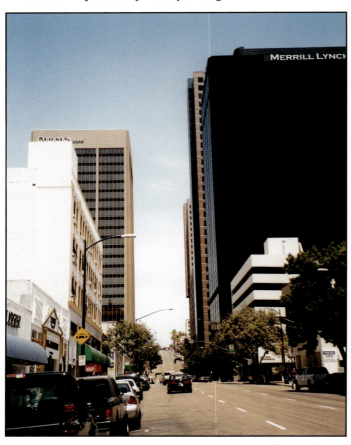

Downtown San Diego.

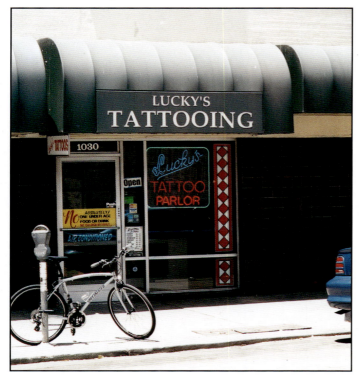

(l. to r.) Vinnie Almanza, Dan Pryor and Luke Wessman.

Lucky's is a very cool shop. It reminds me of Terry Tweed's studio in Portland (I later discovered that Terry helped Dave with the layout). Everything is in its place. Not quite the Terry Tweed version of "everything in its place," mind you, where the edges of every book on the bookshelf are perfectly square with all the other books, but pretty near. The walls are decorated with neatly framed samples of Dave Gibson flash. But coolest of all is the swing-away, gate-like thingy that holds the sheets of laminated flash. Complete with a bench for comfortable browsing, no less. Great idea! The shop is smallish, but the back area opens up into a labyrinth of workstations, each one decorated with classic photos of old-timers and pretty pinups. An elegant, '50s-style layout.

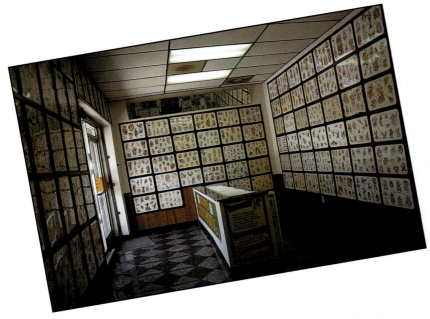

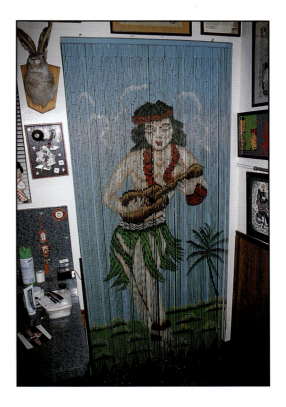

I knew Dave wasn't arriving for another hour, so I took a walk around the neighborhood, being careful not to trip over the drunks. There's a funny balance in downtown San Diego. Seedy but manicured. The sidewalks are clean, the buildings are tidy, but wherever you look there are forlorn souls bumming change or quietly celebrating Roosevelt's inauguration. And plenty of tattoo shops. No kidding, there were five within three blocks. I recognized Masters, of course, the oldest shop in San Diego, but I didn't know the others. Facets on the diamond or weeds in the garden, I hadn't a clue. I wasn't scheduled to visit Masters for a few weeks, but I stopped in to say hello. One of the Lynch brothers, Hiro, was tattooing a young, rather skinny young man. I exchanged pleasantries and headed back to Lucky's.

Dave Gibson was waiting at the door.

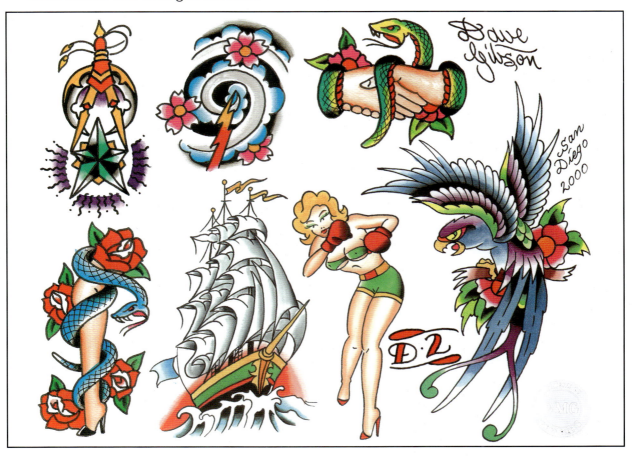

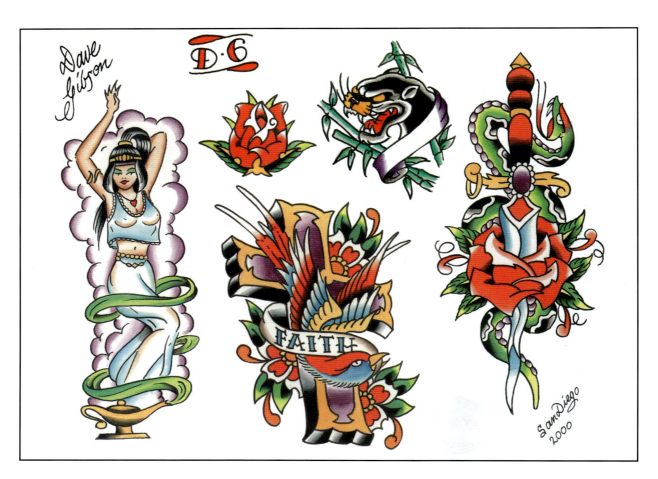

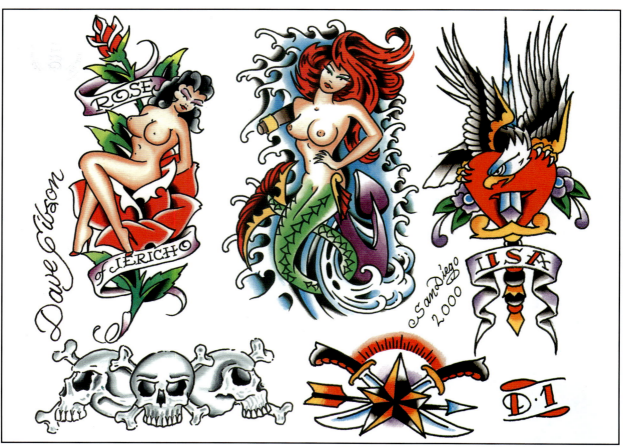

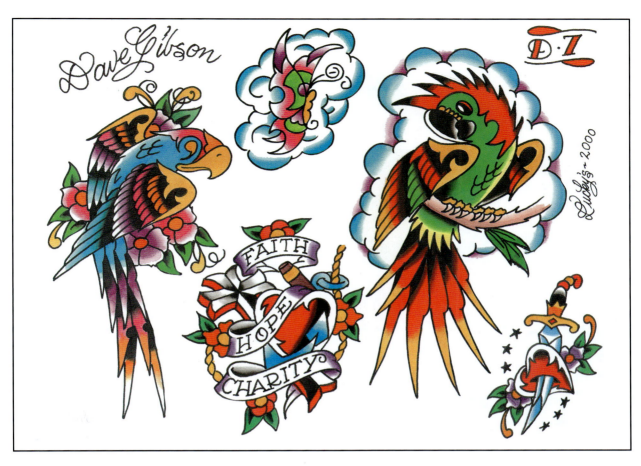

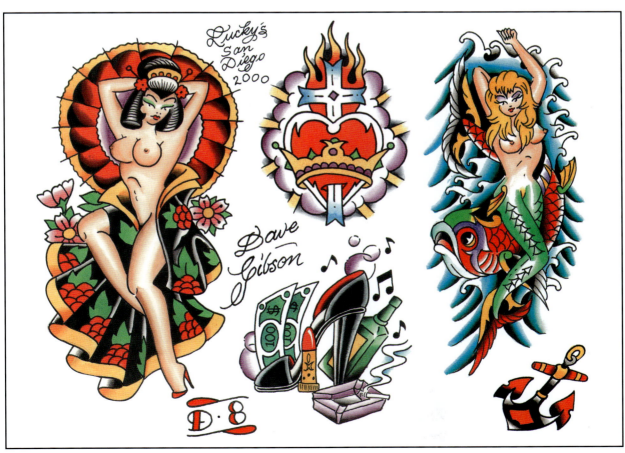

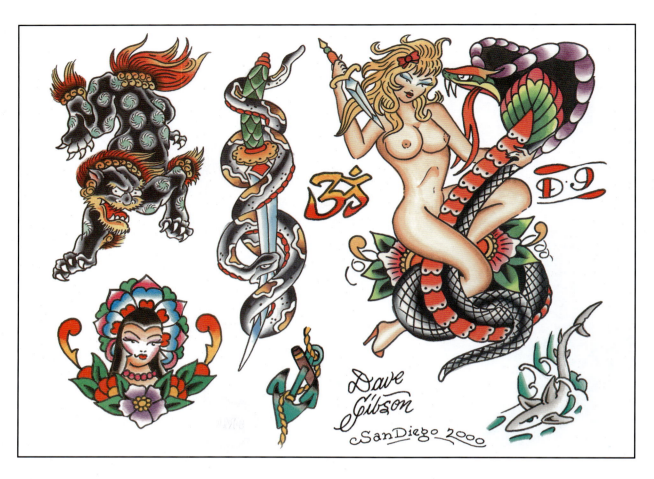

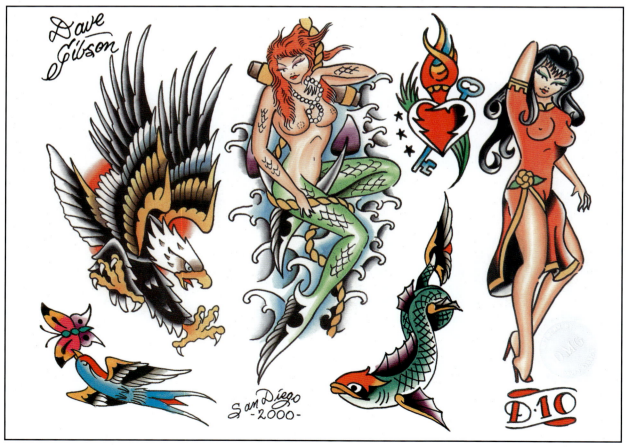

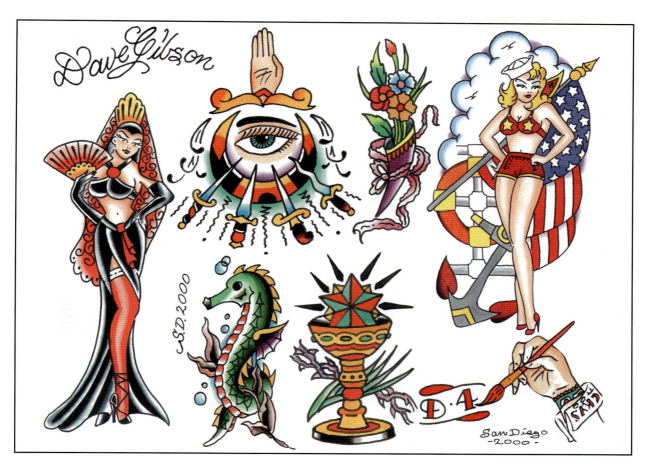

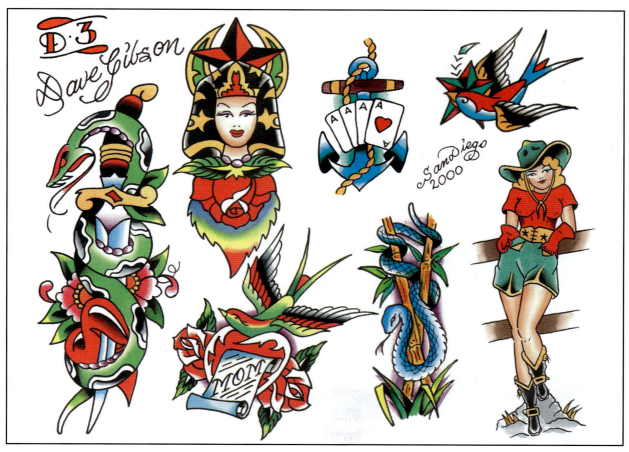

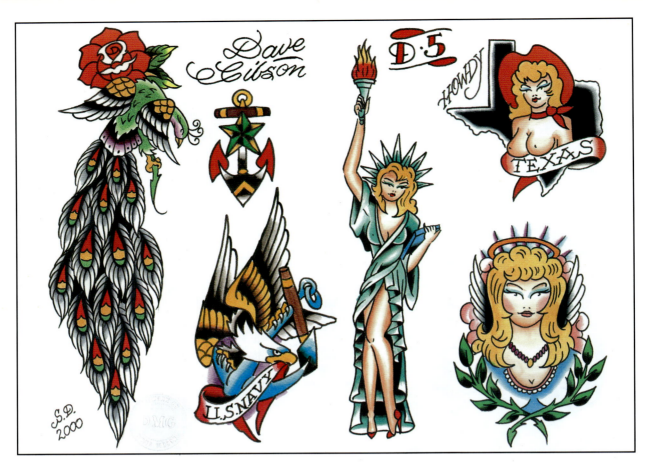

THE ILLUSTRIOUS MR. GIBSON

Never having said two words to Dave before, I recalled the pedal steel guitar I saw in his back room.

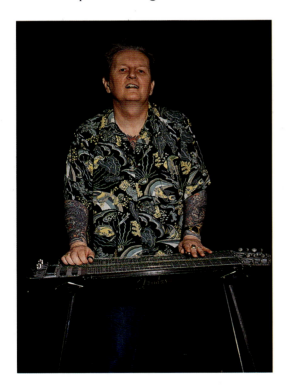

Mr. Dave Gibson and his pedal steel.

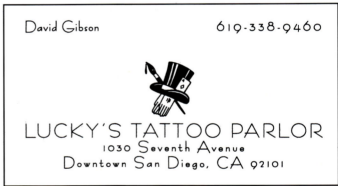

David Gibson   619-338-9460

LUCKY'S TATTOO PARLOR
1030 Seventh Avenue
Downtown San Diego, CA 92101

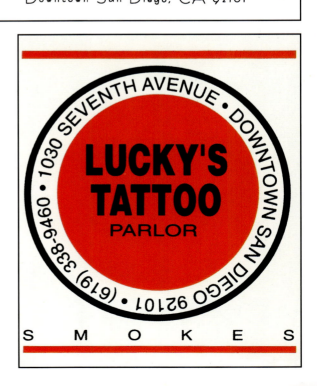

"I play along with the radio when business gets slow," Dave said, smiling.

The next thing I know, Dave's hauling out an old Kentucky Colonel's *Appalachian Swing* album, and I'm promising to send him a copy of the interview with Clarence White from my CBS TV show back in the '70s.

"Who was it that played Dobro for the Colonels?" said Dave, as he scratched his head. "Oh, I remember. Leroy Mack," he recalled, triumphantly.

Not only was Dave a wealth of information about music, he was the perfect person to kick off the book. With a CD of Hank Thompson playing softly in the background, Gibson shared tales of the early years.

Originally from California, Dave left a good-paying job with Bill Loika back at a tiny shop in Deep River, Connecticut, a town of about 4,000. Missing his West Coast roots, Dave returned to California and has been in San Diego for 11 years. He got his first real job from Rex Ross about 22 years ago at a studio in Denver. Before that, Gibson was a "snapper," the sign-painting equivalent of a tattoo scratcher. Having learned sign-painting techniques at L.A Trade Tech, Gibson got customers by placing little ads in the *Penny Saver.*

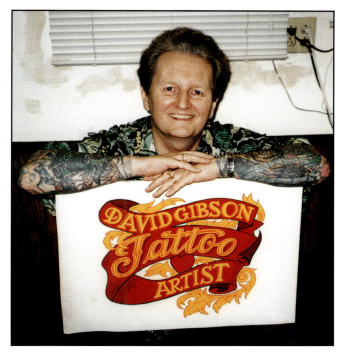

Dave shows off his sign painting handwork.

How did an itinerant sign painter join the extremely strong lineage of legendary tattoo artists? Dave's first teacher, Rex Ross, learned how to tattoo from Bob Shaw and Colonel Todd.

"Rex helped set me up with Colonel Todd to work Bert Grimm's at the Pike in Long Beach. I was there for five years. Rick Walters was there. In fact, he still is! Mark Mahoney was down there too. Todd worked, of course, but on a different shift. I worked the night shift. Todd had another shop on the Pike, and I worked there first for a couple months. And then a position opened up at Bert's, and I got it. Nights for five years.

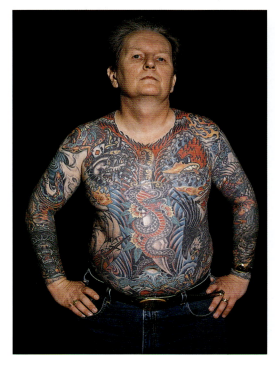

Dave's beautiful tattoos by Bob Roberts.

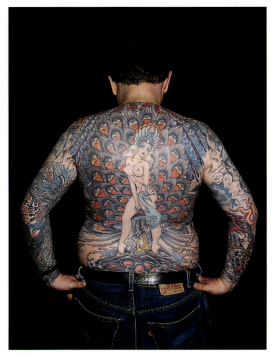

Dave's Bob Roberts backpiece.

"Long Beach didn't have so much military then. We had two battleships stationed there, the *New Jersey* and the *Missouri*. We got our fair share, but not like San Diego. The shop had been there for a long time. It was definitely the most impressive and, by far, the largest shop on the Pike. It had the biggest display. I remember snooping around there in the early-'70s. At that time there were about eight or ten shops, something like that. It was before MTV, before rock stars were sporting tattoos. It was the disco days. The only tattoos I saw back then were on old people. I didn't have friends getting new tattoos. I rarely saw new tattoos on anybody. They were already set in and faded. I would go down there—I wasn't getting any tattoos. I was enthralled with the artwork. The flash turned me on. It wasn't airbrushed. How did they do that? I have a piece of old Bert Grimm flash up on the wall. I rescued it out of the trash.

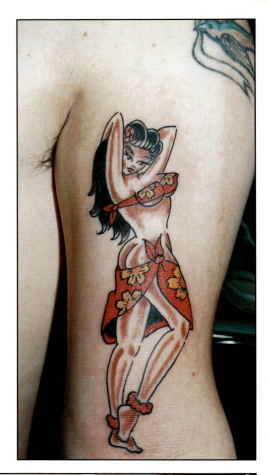

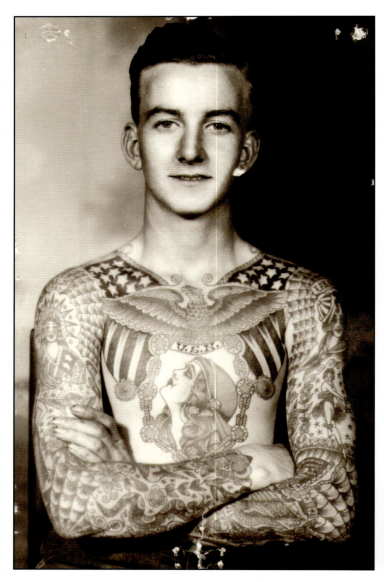

Bob Shaw tattooed by Bert Grimm in St. Louis, Missouri, 1940s.
Photo courtesy of Tattoo Archive.

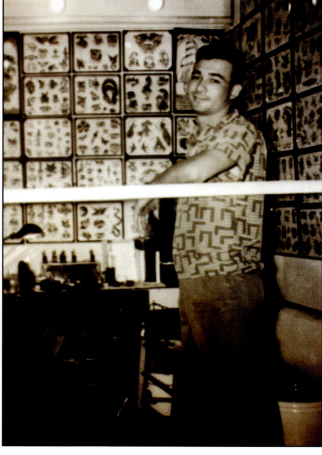

Col. W.L. Todd in his Clarksville, Tennessee, shop, 1950s.
Photo courtesy of Tattoo Archive.

16

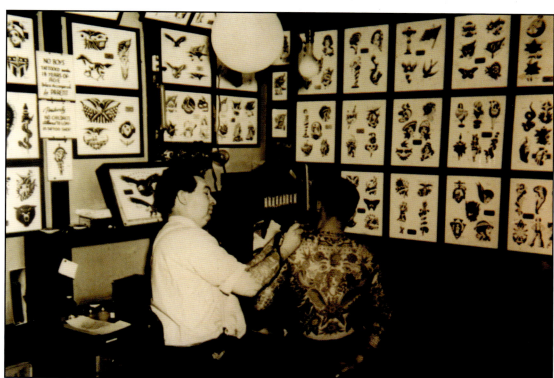

Bert Grimm tattooing in St. Louis, Missouri, 1940s. *Photo courtesy of Tattoo Archive.*

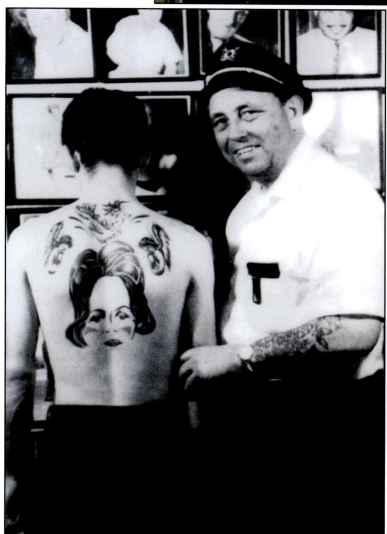

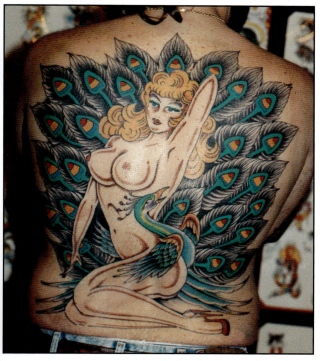

Doc Webb showing his tattooing, San Diego, Calfornia, 1960s. *Photo courtesy of Tattoo Archive.*

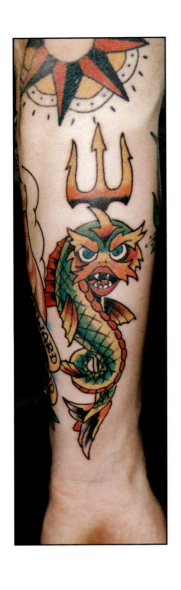

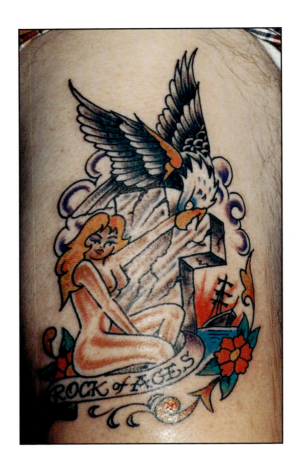

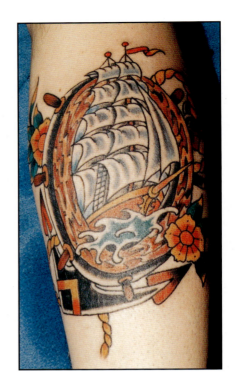

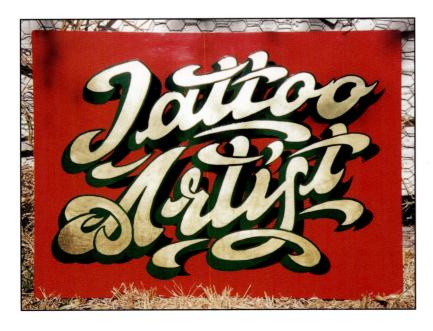

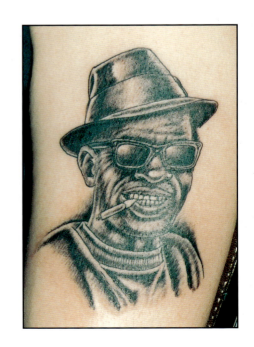

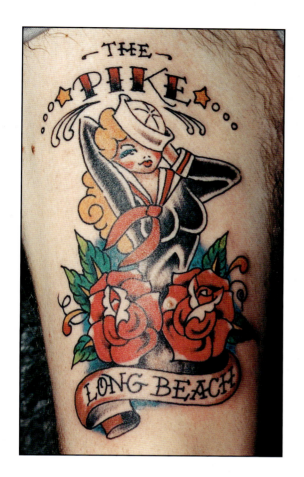

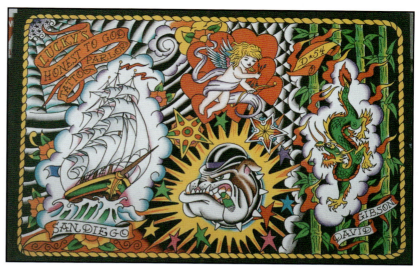

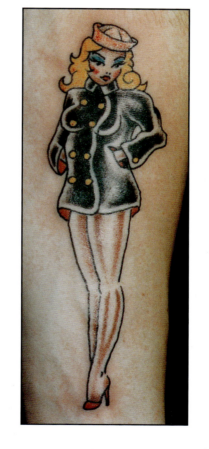

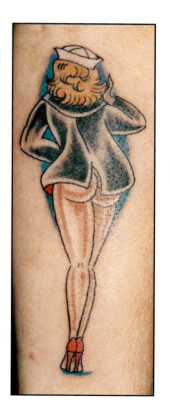

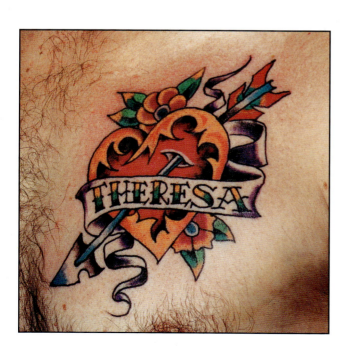

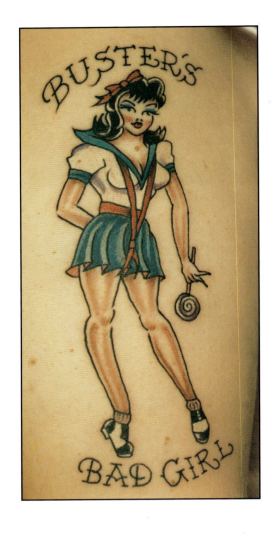

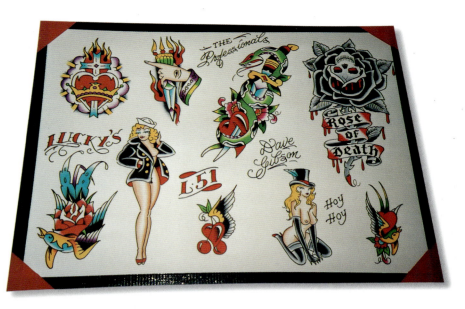

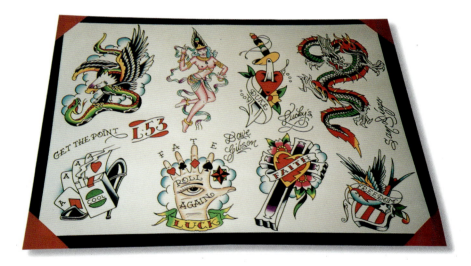

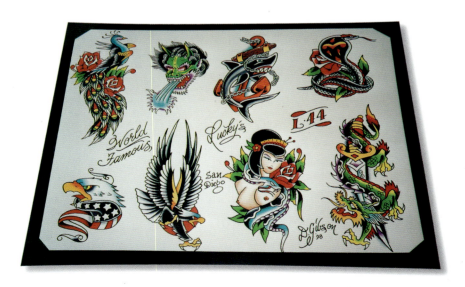

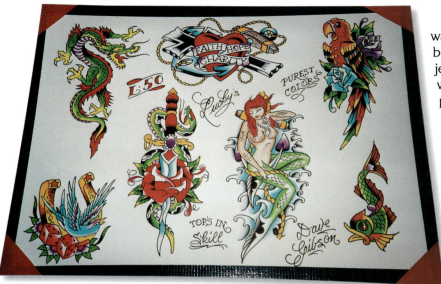

"In 1978 or 1979, I came down to San Diego on a little expedition and parked my car at the train station. When I got home, I had about 12 business cards from 12 different shops. All within walking distance. And that was before you got to the numbered streets. There's India, Columbia, State Street—maybe about ten blocks. That's where the tattoo shops were. Doc Webb was on Fourth Avenue. That was about as far as anyone went. He was pretty much out of the real hub back then. I remember seeing shops literally next door to each other. You would walk out of one shop next door to another one. They were all downtown. They were all busy. Everybody knew to go downtown to get a tattoo.

"Then the city came in and rebuilt downtown. They shoved everybody out from where they were working. They tore down the buildings. There used to be arcades and stuff down there. All fun stuff. It's all spread out anymore. Now there's tattoo shops in every tiny little town. It used to be that a tattoo was a souvenir you brought back from somewhere else, not just walk down to the corner.

"Back then, driving from Gardena to San Diego—there were tattoo shops in Long Beach. I didn't know of any in Orange County. I think Bert Grimm had one there for awhile. Bob Shaw put it together for him, just to give him something to do. I think it was in Santa Ana.

"As far I knew, there were shops in the San Fernando Valley and downtown Los Angeles. There was one that didn't last very long in San Pedro, in the same era. Then Long Beach and San Diego. That's all I knew of. I used to visit the library and go through the Yellow Pages to see where I could find a tattoo shop. I wanted to go and investigate. Back then, there wasn't much literature on it. I was just reading an article by Ed Hardy where he

was saying in the '50s there were only four books in English published on the subject of tattooing. It pretty much stayed that way up until the '70s. Then some bits and pieces started coming out. *Easyrider* magazines started featuring tattooing here and there. You'd see tattoos in biker publications. But there sure wasn't exposure like it is now.

"To me, the mystery of tattooing is gone. It used to be, if you'd go in and ask questions, they'd basically tell you to get the hell out. They weren't worried about you coming back or telling your friends they were rude or anything. I got the bum's rush, basically. There was one old-timer—I don't know what his name was—he sat and talked to me for a while. It was a plethora of information just to have somebody respond. I asked him, 'How do you learn?' He said, 'Go up to Northern California to one of those little farm communities and tattoo some lettuce pickers up there.' Really, that was his advice to me. You get to practice. Hardworking people really love tattoos. They won't have any money. And, oddly enough, that's basically what I'm looking for here in San Diego: Hardworking people who like tattoos."

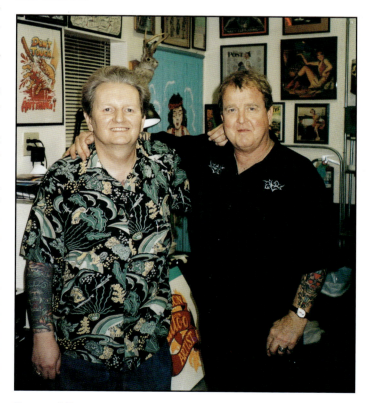

Dave and Baxter.

DANIELLE OBEROSLER
& ROBERT ATKINSON
MELROSE TATTOO, HOLLYWOOD

Melrose Avenue rocks! Located in famous "Hollyweird," this ten-block fashion sideshow of hip shops and trendy restaurants is about 30 minutes from home. Acknowledged as a Mecca for people-watching, on weekends the sidewalks of Melrose Avenue host a bountiful barrage of startled starlets and bulimic nymphets teetering on eight-inch heels, while their boyfriends do their best James Dean. Then, of course, there are the weekend road warriors with their spotless $50,000 Harleys parked in front of the local burger barn. Did I mention the hordes of tourists with their cameras? Whatever your pleasure, there are probably more shoe showrooms, bustier emporiums, and condom shops on this five-furlong slice of real estate than anywhere else in Los Angeles.

And perched above the mayhem reside my dear friends Robert Atkinson and Danielle Oberosler. Robert I met when my sons Jesse and Riley worked just up the street at Body Electric with Pote Seyler. Those dudes split to the four corners, but Robert keeps the tattoo tradition alive and kicking at Melrose Tattoo. Sure, Spotlight is a couple miles east, but that's another part of town, as far as I'm concerned, and no-where near this particular pandering pulse of plentiful pulchritude.

Robert Atkinson.

RAMBLIN' ROBERT

Never content to settle in one place, Robert Atkinson travels a lot. Like many an itinerant artist, Robert divides his time among Melrose Tattoo, Eternal Art in Santa Clarita, and Tattoo Deluxe in San Pedro, plus a private studio. And, just so he doesn't get bored, Robert flies to Europe every so often to work with Greg Orie at Dragon Tattoo in Holland and his friend Henning Jorgenson at Royal Tattoo in Helsingor, Denmark.

I've kept in touch with Robert through my magazine, but I haven't seen him in the flesh for quite some time. He sends me photos every few months, so I know he's doing fine, but our paths haven't crossed for a few years. By the way, I can always spot Robert's tattoos. It's his trademark refinement of technique and line. Clean graphics, solid composition, bright colors. Robert is a rock-solid artist.

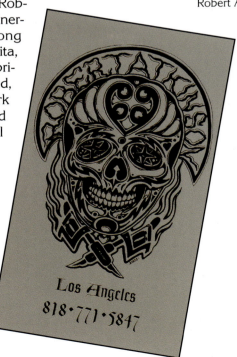

Los Angeles
818·771·5847

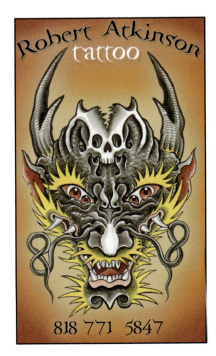

Robert Atkinson
tattoo

818 771 5847

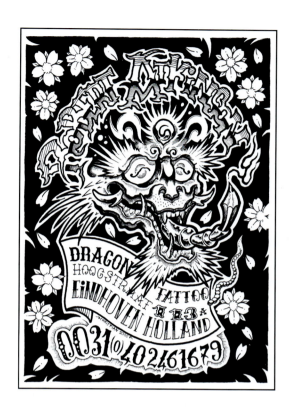

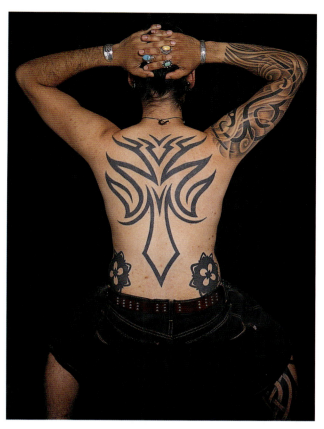

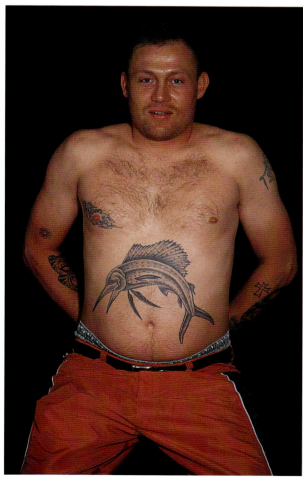

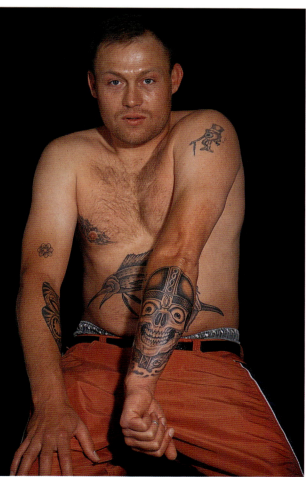

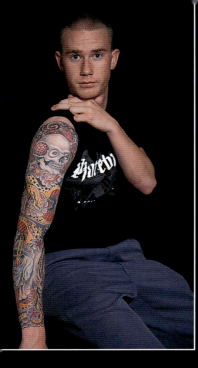
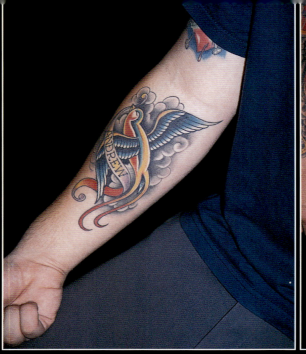
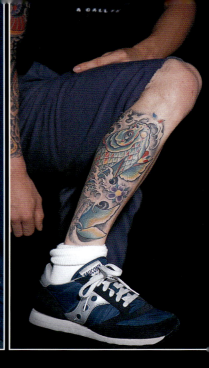
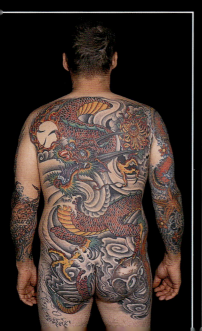
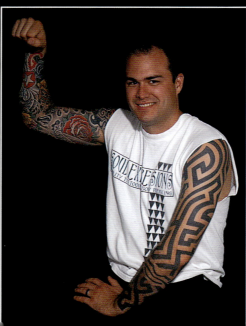
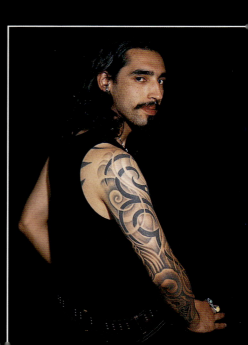

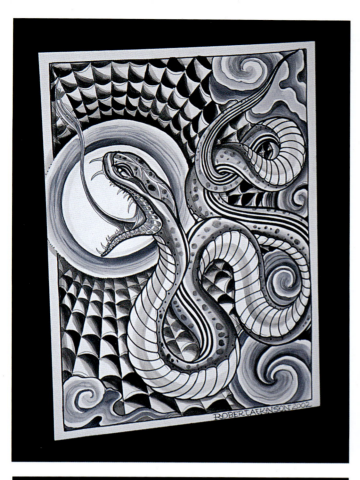

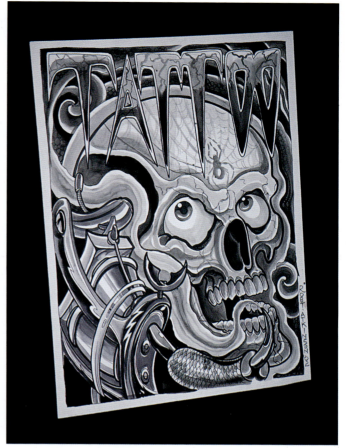

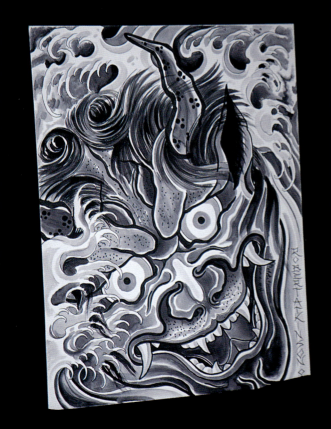

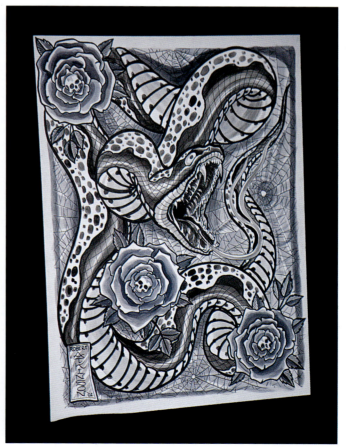

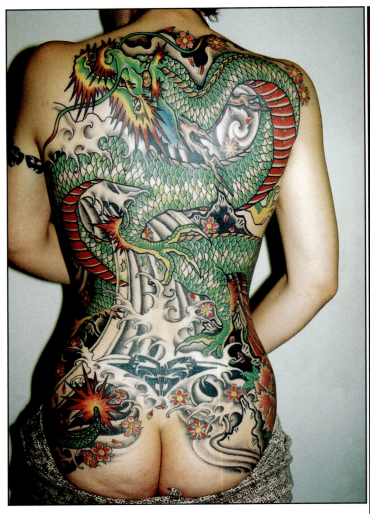

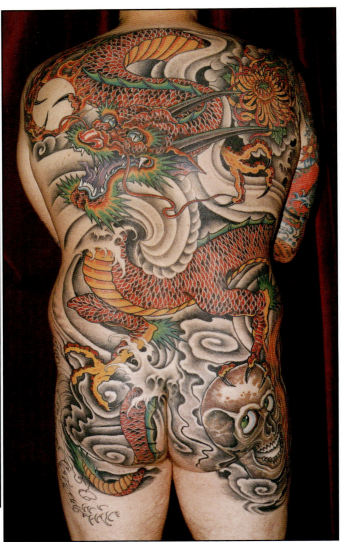

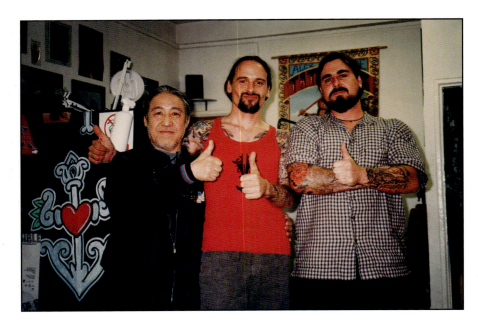

Robert with Horiyoshi III (l.) and
Mick at Into You in London, 1996.

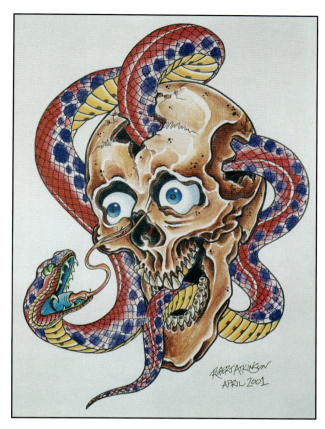

Robert's flash from 2001.

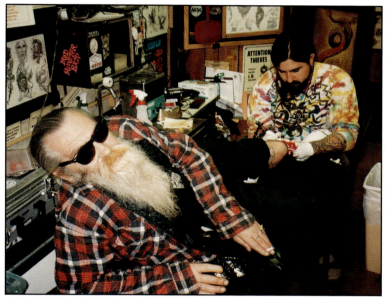

Tattooing Rick Walters at Bert Grimm's, Long Beach, 1997.

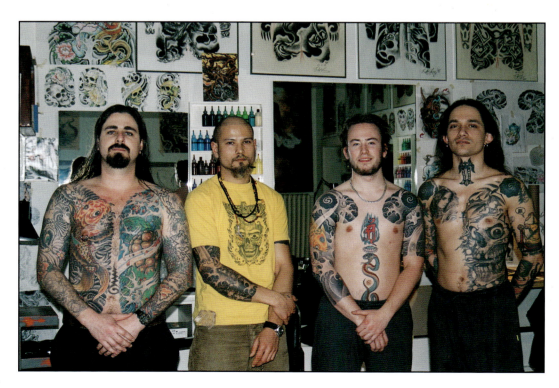

(l. to r.) Robert, Rinzing, Wido, and Filp Leu at Filip's shop in Lausanne, Switzerland, 2001.

A PAL OF MINE

I met Danielle Oberosler when she worked at Art and Soul, Erika Stanley's shop on Robertson in West L.A.. Since then, Danielle has proven to be both an excellent artist and talented writer. Penning the column *Spotlight* for SKIN & INK, Dani keeps tabs on the world's emerging and sometimes overlooked tattoo shops from Aspen to Amsterdam. People respond well to Danielle's outgoing personality. She digs up stories other people can't. Chalk it up to her winning smile, but I think her tattoos have something to do with it. In a world of inflated egos, it doesn't hurt that the reporter is a damn good artist in her own right. Tattooers can be snobbish, and unless you know how to deal, they won't give you the time of day. Like the time I saw a neophyte writer ask an old-timer what he used to mix his inks.

"Piss and treacle," was the answer. The journalist, of course, enthusiastically jotted the info down in his notebook. This wouldn't happen the Danielle. She knows her treacle.

By the way, Danielle has come to my rescue more than once, and when I mentioned to a couple of big-name hotshops and that Danielle was going to be included in this book, they nodded and said, "She does righteous work." What, no sexist remarks? Man, these tattoo artists are becoming more enlightened all the time.

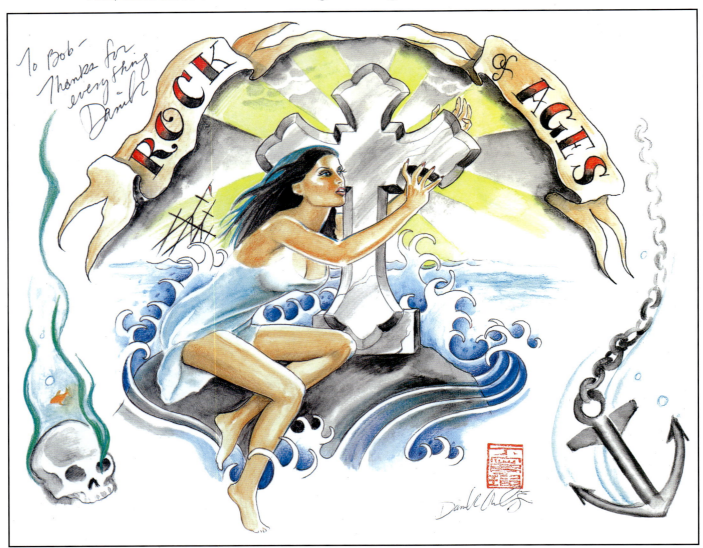

Examples of Danielle's flash.

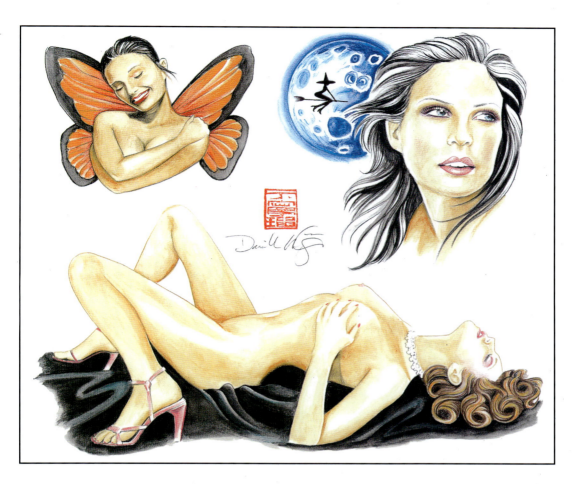

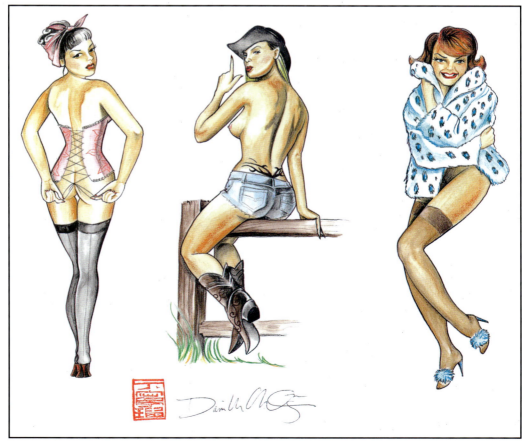

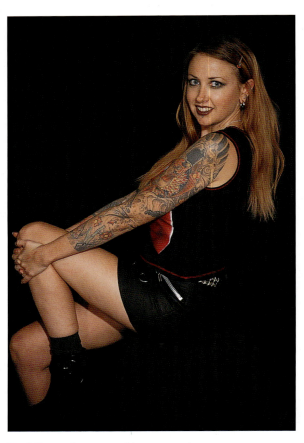

Danielle emulates one of her saucy pinups.

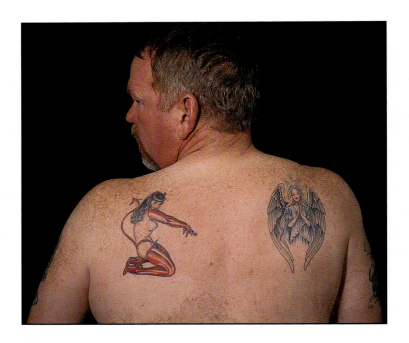

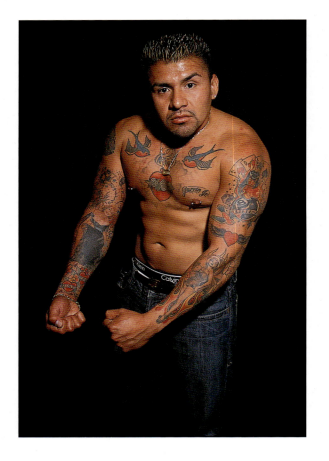

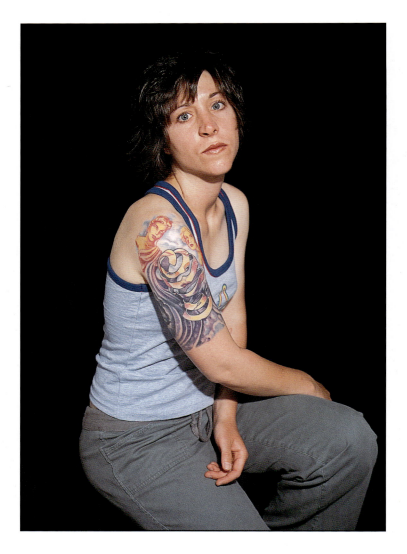

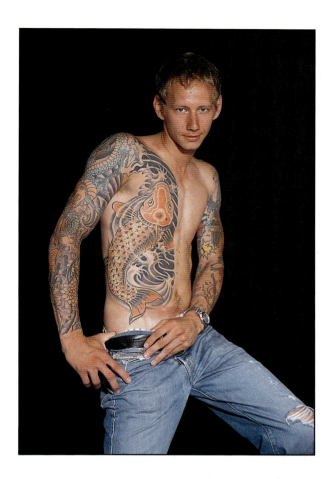
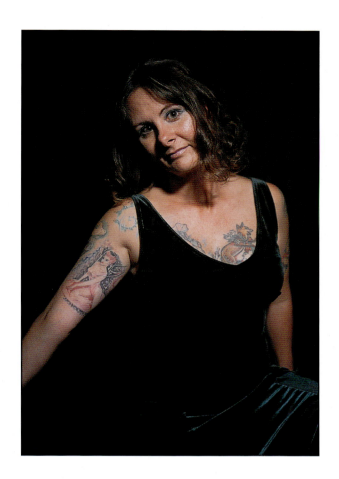
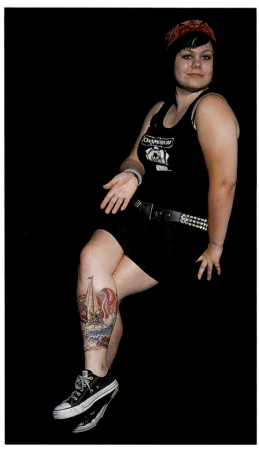
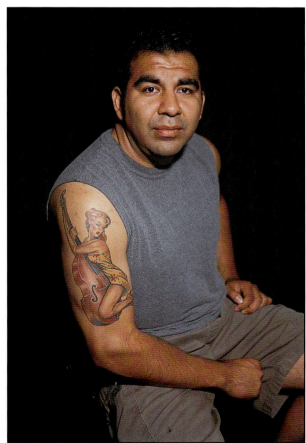

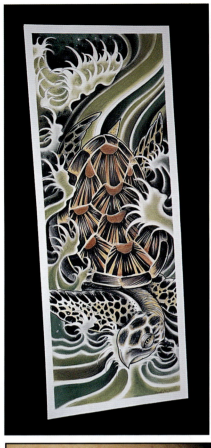

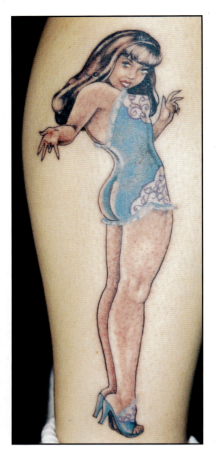

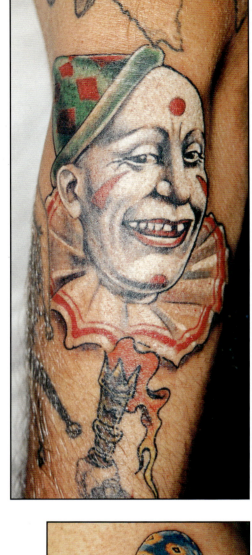

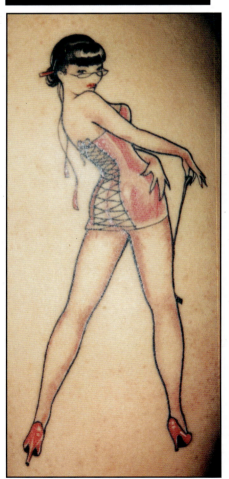

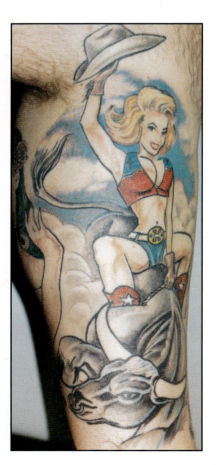

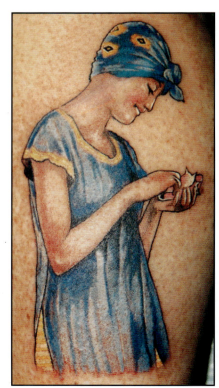

ON TOP OF THE WORLD

I wished I'd hired a sherpa to help me up the stairs at 7661½ Melrose. Weighted down with cameras, a tripod and an aluminum ladder, I looked like a one-man band. But I made it, and even though the place is extremely small, it's neat and efficient. I was especially glad to see Robert, of course. It had been way too long. Funny, we picked up our conversation where we left off some four years ago. It was fun to hear about his adventures in Lausanne with the Leu Family Iron. In homage to mountainous Switzerland, we climbed up a rickety wrought-iron ladder to converse on the rooftop.

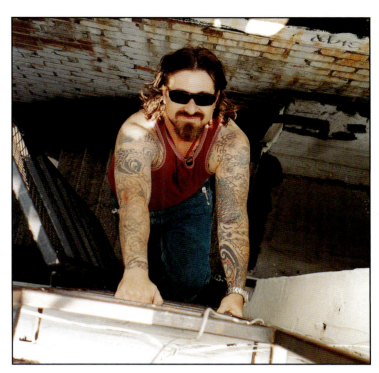

Robert on the ladder.

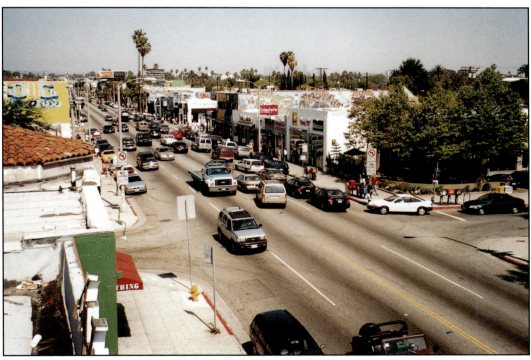

Bird's eye view of Melrose Avenue.

"You can get a great photograph of the street from here," Robert assured me.

After we climbed back down, the clients began to show. Danielle coordinated the shoot and needled us unmercifully. Although she's been branching out with her Tattoo Lady product line, Danielle has been churning out a lot of good work and establishing herself as one of L.A.'s better pinup artists. It's good to see she's working with Robert for a few hours each week. I got a kick out of their sarcastic banter. The perfect attitude on a blazing-hot Southern California afternoon.

SHANNON O'SULLIVAN
SHANGRI-LA TATTOO, ALTADENA

Shannon O'Sullivan has worked out of her tie-dyed, macraméd, '60s-style tattoo shop for the last six years. Tucked away in a quiet section of Altadena, five minutes from my house, Shangri-la is more like a retro coffeehouse than a tattoo studio. Lots of tapestries, scented candles, and jeweled mirrors inhabit every space and countertop. The backyard is like a shrine. Perfect for parties, flowered trellises section off secret pathways and cozy conversation pits. Plump little Buddhas, bunny rabbits, and terra-cotta Krishnas poke their heads from behind hand-painted flowerpots and untamed ivy. The perfect lair for butterflies and dragons.

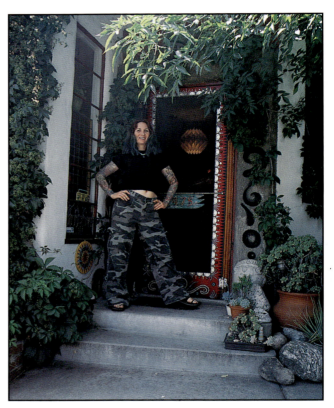

Shannon O'Sullivan.

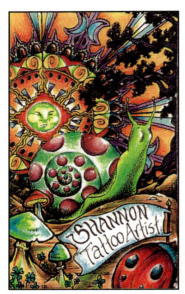

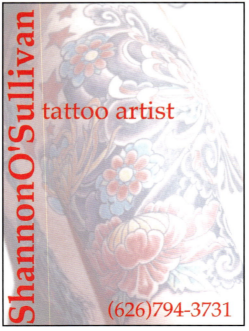

ShannonO'Sullivan

tattoo artist

(626)794-3731

THE VALLEY GIRL

I met Shannon about eight years ago. I think it was at Body Electric. She was making the rounds, getting her daily whiff of green soap. Apprenticing briefly with Tattoo Mike in the early-'90s, Shannon has plied the trade nearly 12 years, but started making money as an artist when she was 15. You know those hand-painted footballs and basketballs that high schools put in their trophy cases when they win a championship? Shannon was the school's head trophy-ball painter. She also did photographic copies of album covers on the backs of denim jackets for $200 a pop. "Hey, I did one or two a month," she smiles. After high school, Shannon studied at Parson's School of Design and, after that, Art Center. "I come from a family of artists, musicians and scientists. My father was always supportive about my being an artist," she recalls. "In fact, he used to live with the famous tattooist Cap Szumski. Cap lived at my dad's ranch out in Canyon Country and tattooed Dad extensively. I have a very special family. My dad knew tattoo artists can make good money, and he was the one that suggested I give it a try."

Overnight, Shannon became a tattoo junkie, checking out the local scene, especially Tattoo Mike's, right around the corner from her house in Sunland/Tujunga. Mike welcomed Shannon and paid her to color in his old biker flash—wizards, peacocks, and grim reapers.

"I lived, breathed and ate tattooing. I checked out everything I could get my hands on. There was very little available. Up until then, it was *Easyrider* magazines, and that was about it. Then the first *Skin Art* came out. I saw what Jill Jordan and Guy Aitchison were doing. It was like they had unlocked the code."

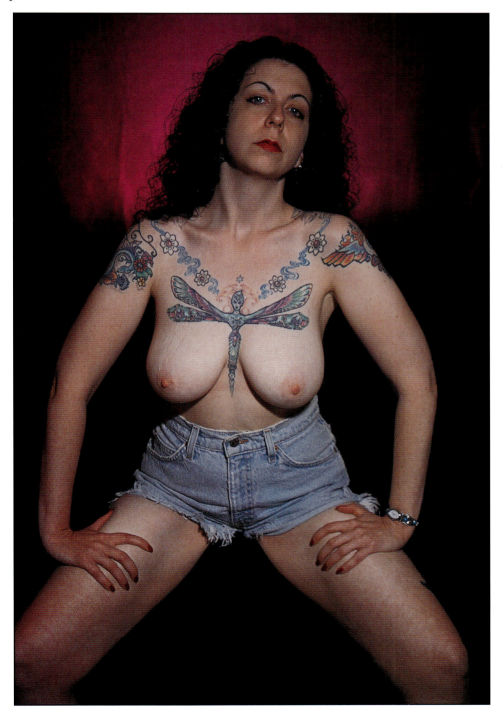

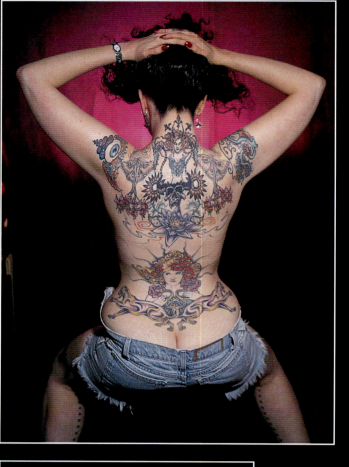
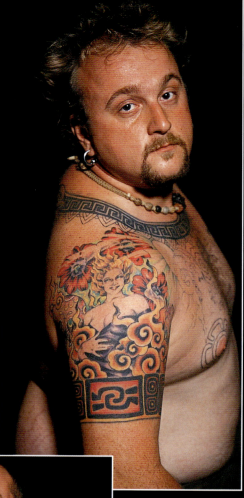
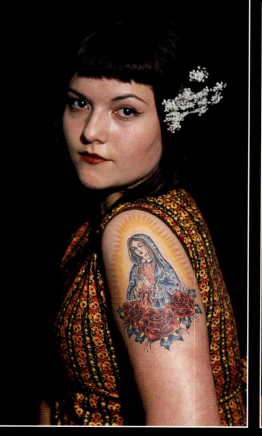
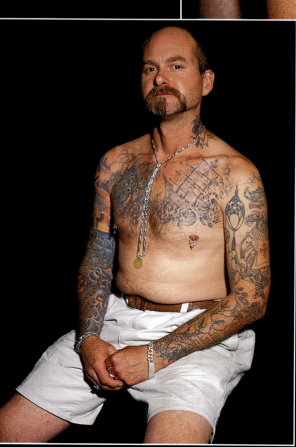

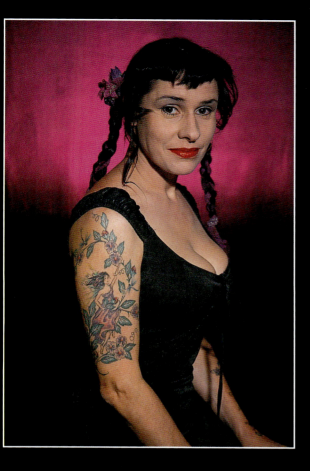
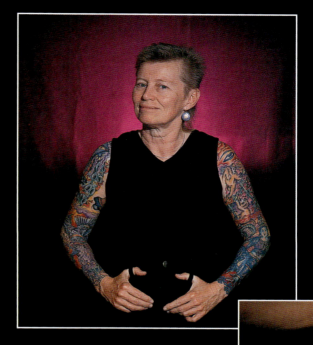
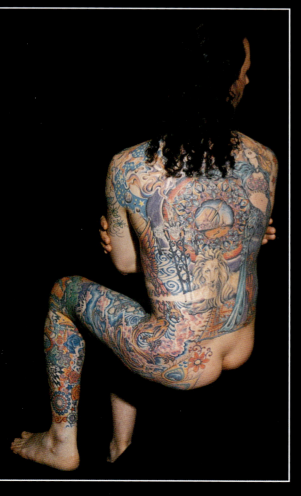
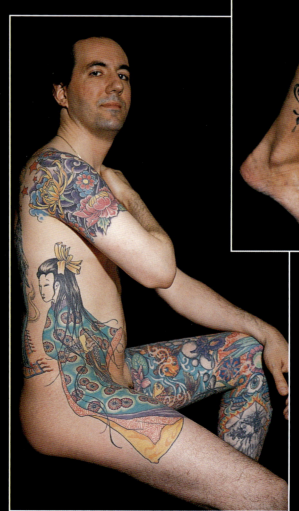

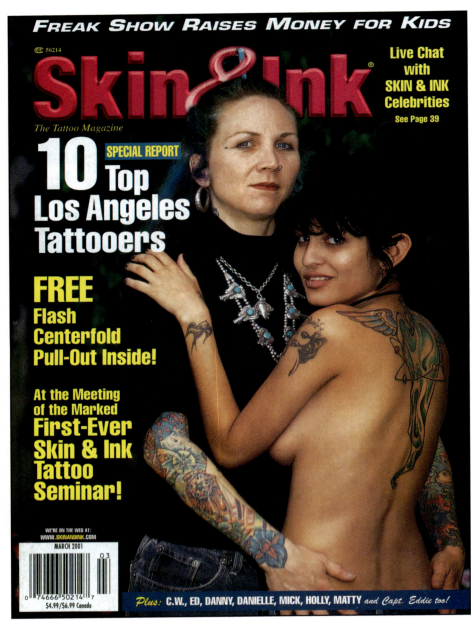

Receiving more phone calls than any other artist after being featured in SKIN & INK's *L.A.'s Ten Top Tattooists* issue, Shannon has always shunned the mainstream, choosing instead to share her skills with a dedicated following of poets, musicians, homemakers, and free thinkers. As I was setting up my lights for the photo-shoot, everyone who came through the door was greeted with a hoot and a hug. It was the same selfless, positive energy I've experienced before with Shannon. The same magnetic, Earth-mother spirit that captures a person's essence and turns it into a tattoo—the warmth and friendliness that keeps her customers and friends coming back again and again to that mystical space at the edge of the beautiful San Gabriel mountains.

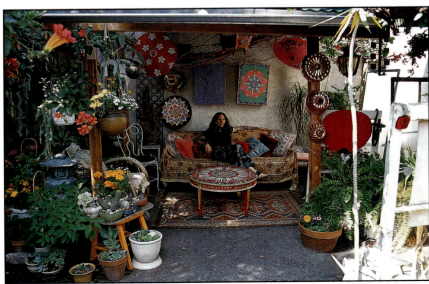

Shannon in her garden.

MIKE PIKE &
JOJO ACKERMANN
PSYCHO CITY TATTOOING, LANCASTER

You think Shannon O'Sullivan is out of the mainstream; that's nothing compared to Mike Pike and Jojo Ackermann. Mike's shop, Psycho City, is located at the virtual gateway to the Mojave desert, smack dab in the middle of the Antelope Valley, about three miles past where Jesus lost his shoes. In fact, when you turn off the 5 and go east on the 14 toward Lancaster, it's moonscape time. Except for the ticky-tack bedroom communities sprouting out of the sandy fields, there's nothing but tumbleweeds. Yup, once the home of dehydrated lizards and a couple land turtles, this beatific badlands has been victimized by the urban sprawl of orange-tiled roofs, built-in dishwashers and central air.

But beyond the tracts, beyond the electric traffic lights, beyond the smoke and chaos of the big city, the two-lane blacktop cuts through some pretty amazing real estate. It's not often I take this back way to Las Vegas, just over the hill from the manicured lawns and Craftsman homes of old Pasadena. But I doggedly pressed on through the heat, past the plastic neighborhoods, past the Pearblossom cutoff, past the Lamont "Monty" Odett scenic view site to an area so remote, it doesn't even have street names. It has letters like A, B and C. In fact, when I spotted D Street, I knew I was getting close. Psycho City is on I street, just a few consonants away.

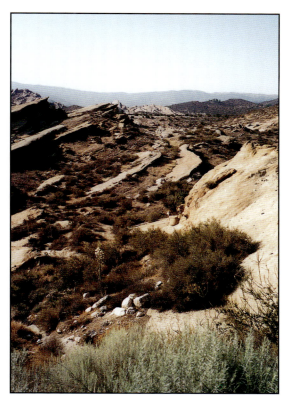

The beautiful countryside on the way to Lancaster.

THE LOCAL HOT SPOT

Sure, the car radio went crazy for a while, and I forgot to bring bottled water, but it's beautiful, and time flew by. In fact, when I spotted Psycho City, I was 20 minutes early. It had only taken an hour. So, after recharging my batteries with a little fast-food soda pop, I cruised across the street, slid in behind a couple tricked-out choppers and unpacked. Once inside, it was sensory overload. A virtual oasis of heavy metal, revved-up customers, and peanut sauce. Mike's restaurant buddy, Surat "Sam" Lertpiriyapong, had prepared a massive Thai buffet—big, aluminum trays of roasted chicken, fried rice, spicy beef salad, chicken chow mein and tubs of special sauce. Plus, in all my previous *Road Trips*, I can't remember a bigger turn-out. There was a line out the door. It was wall-to-wall back- and chestpieces. Everyone had major ink. Solid work. World-class work.

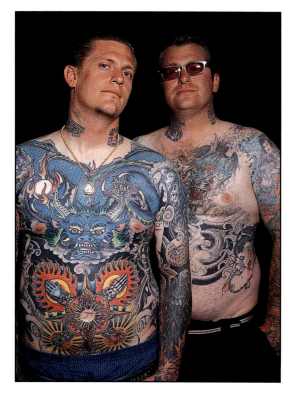

Jojo Ackerman and Mike Pike (wearing shades).

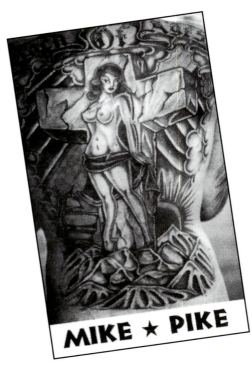

MIKE ★ PIKE

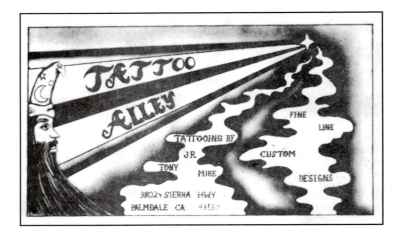

TATTOO ALLEY

FINE LINE

TATTOOING BY
JR CUSTOM
TONY MIKE DESIGNS

38024 SIERRA HWY
PALMDALE CA 93550

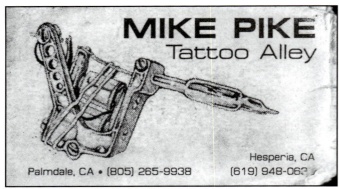

MIKE PIKE
Tattoo Alley

Hesperia, CA
Palmdale, CA • (805) 265-9938   (619) 948-063_

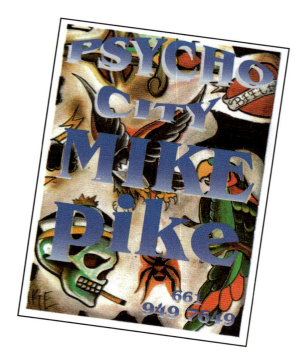

PSYCHO CITY MIKE Pike

661 949 7649

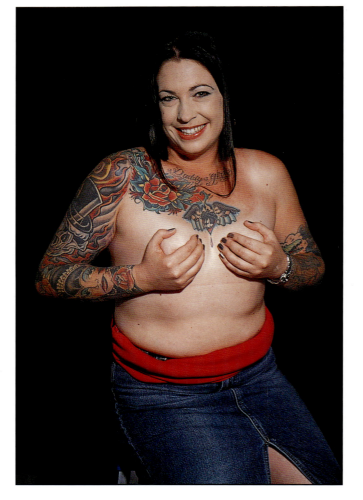

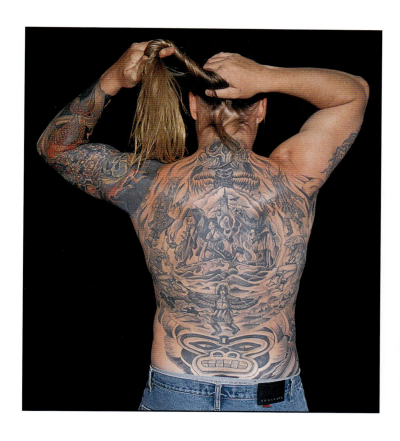

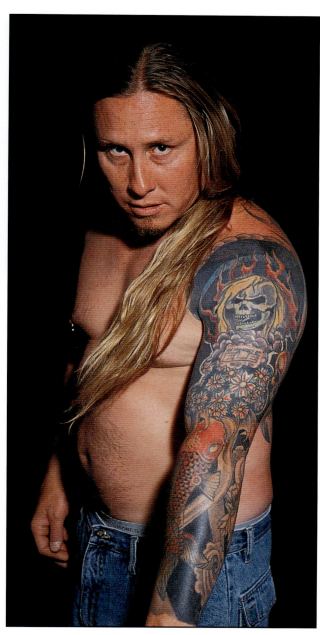

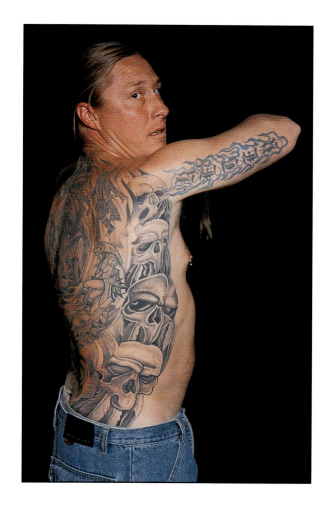

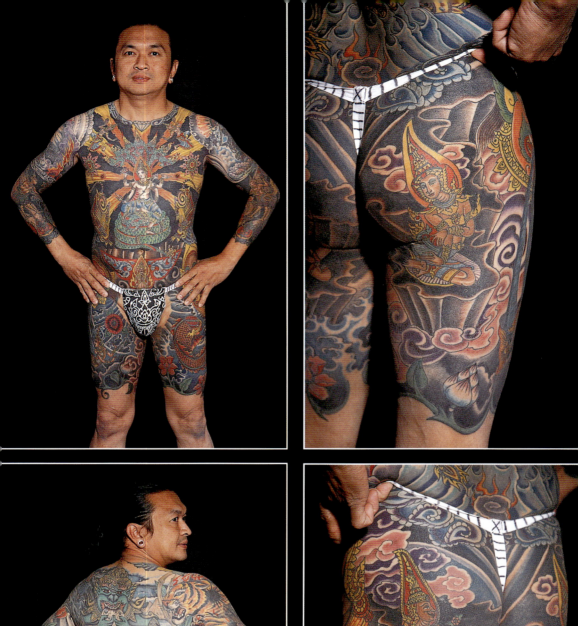
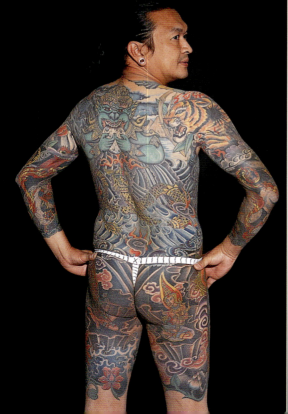
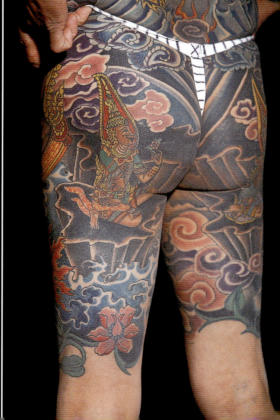

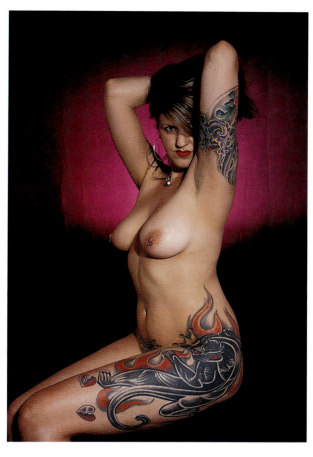 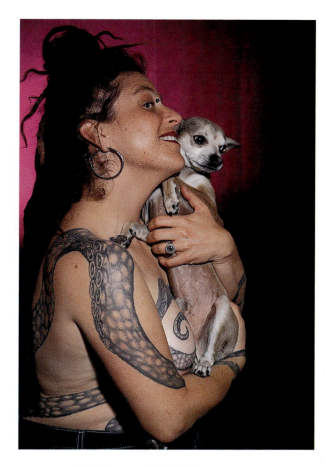

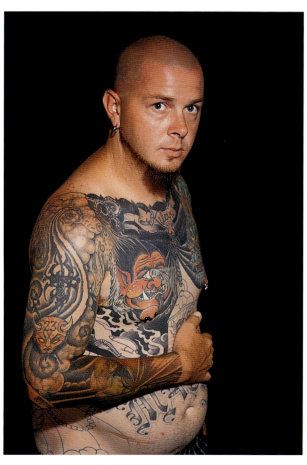 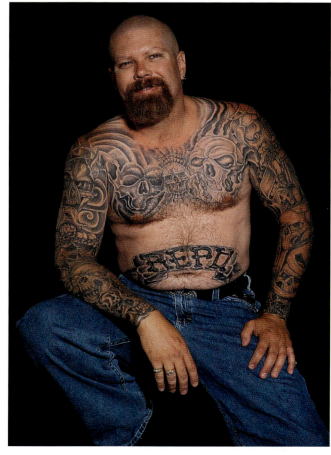

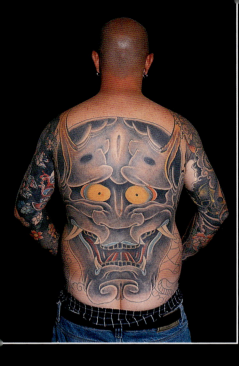
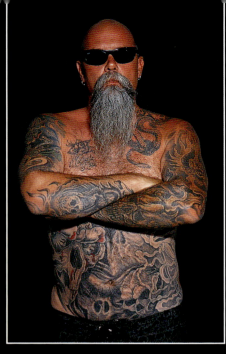
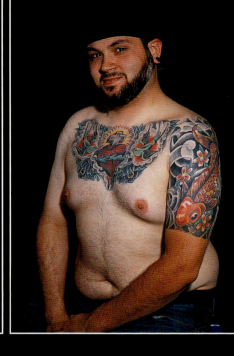
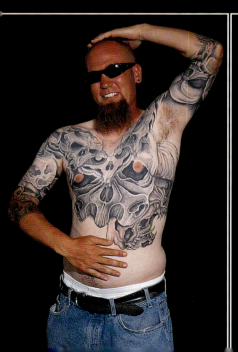
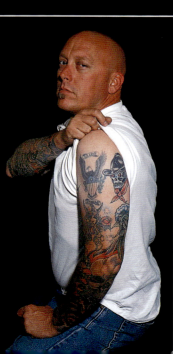
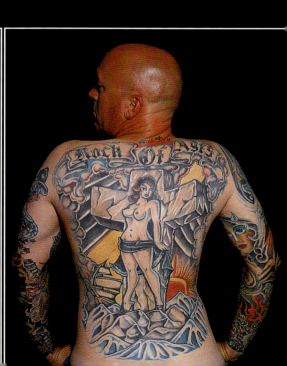

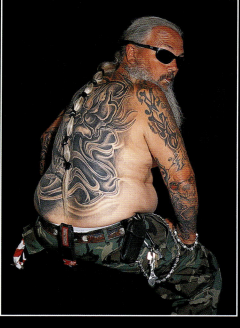
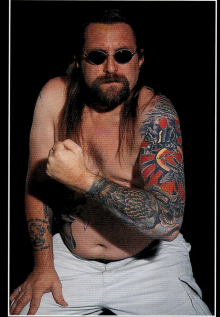
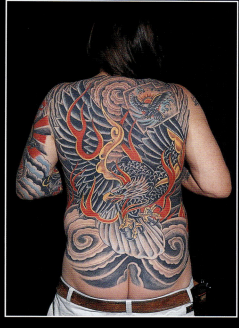

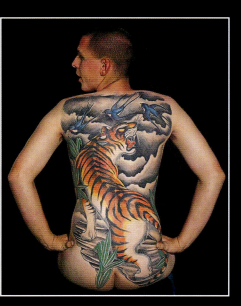
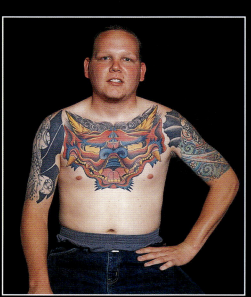
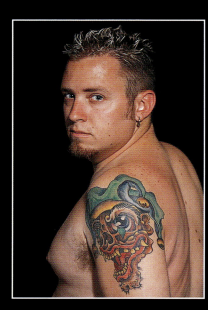

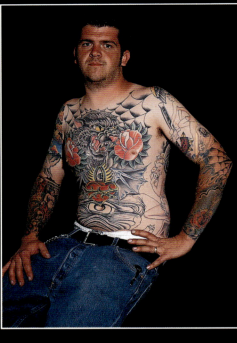
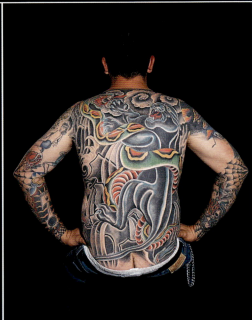
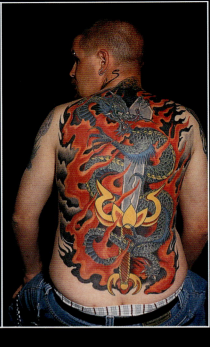
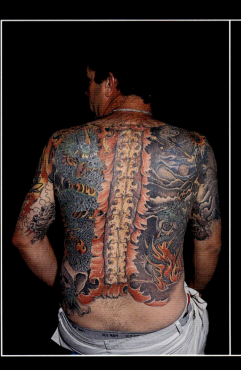
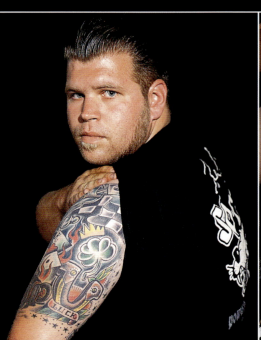
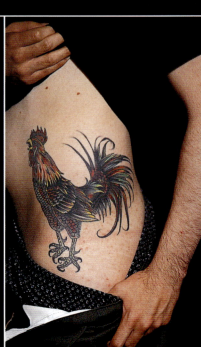

46

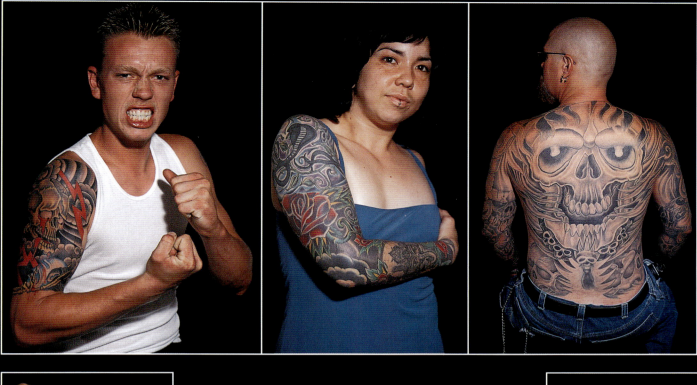

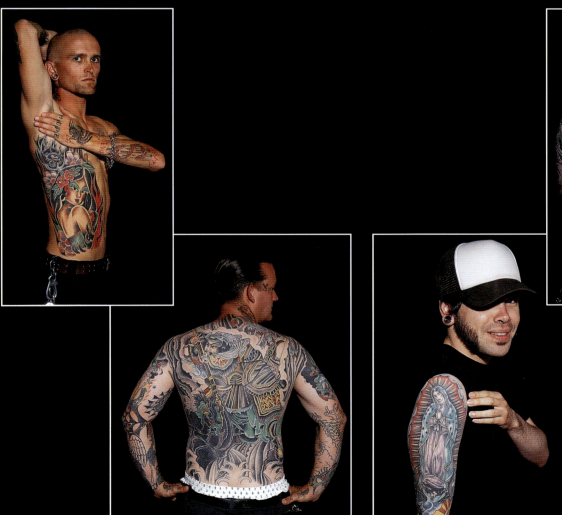

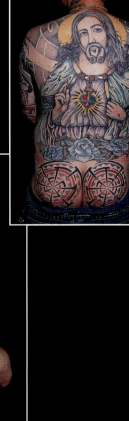

As for my pals Mike and Jojo, legend has it that Mike Pike was hatched in an autoclave. He virtually grew up in his dad J.R. Grove's shop, Tattoo Alley, in Palmdale. Mike started tattooing at eight and did his first backpiece when he was 14! Jojo was born and bred in Lancaster, hanging out at Tattoo Alley when he was 14. Jojo has only worked at one shop, Psycho City, for the last ten years.

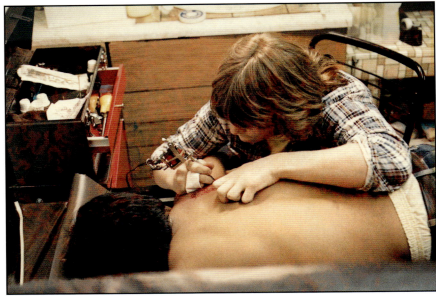

Young Mike at 13, tattooing Leo Sandaval, 1983 (look, no gloves!).

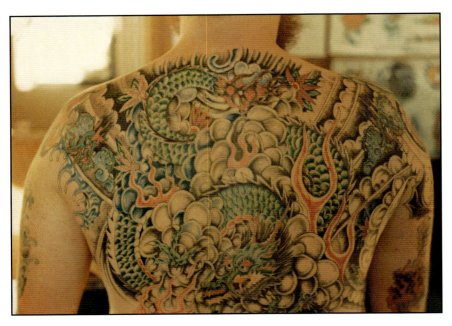

Mike's first backpiece at age 14, 1984.

For sure, Lancaster is remote and off the beaten path. But that's not a bad thing. Mike Pike, his crew and his customers don't take a backseat to the big city. The tattoos are as vital, dynamic, and mainstream as anything I've seen by the best in America or Europe. Yes, Lancaster is but a dot on the map, but you won't see small-town ink. This is not the home of wizards or Tazmanian devils. This is the home of big-city bold. Backs and shoulders and chests. You know as well as I, people don't commit to major tattoo work unless they're inspired. So, you sheiks and sheikettes, looking for some high-desert ink? It's time to steer your camel toward exotic Lancaster and quench your thirst at the virtual oasis called Psycho City.

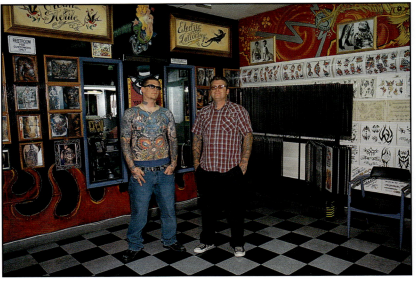

Jojo and Mike.

BOB ROBERTS
SPOTLIGHT TATTOO, HOLLYWOOD

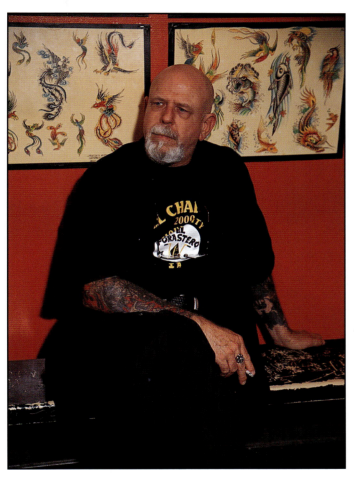

Bob Roberts.

The word is out, it's all about real estate. An unmarked chest. A virgin back. Terrific real estate. But there's nothing to equal the real estate of a forearm; a naked, unblemished, nontattooed forearm. That's primo property. To my way of thinking, it's the most important place to wear a tattoo. Everyone can see it. Short sleeves? No problem. You look at it every day of your life. Wash your hands—it's there. Button your fly—it's there. Cross your arms—it's there. So be smart. Don't give your best real estate to some scratcher or second-rate poser. Be patient. Wait for the best.

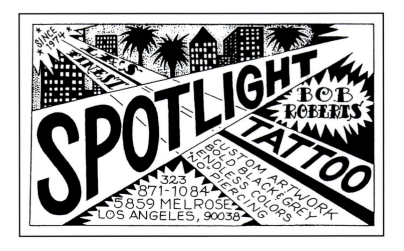

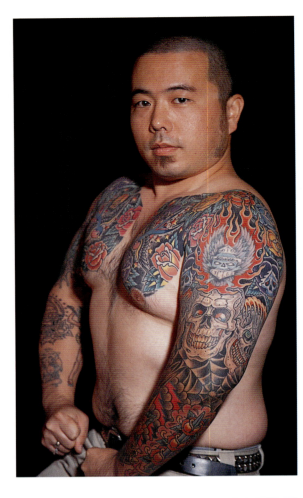

I held out for years. I took my time and considered the choices carefully. Did I go the celebrity route? After all, how cool would it be to say, "Glad you like it. It's a Sailor Jerry Collins." He's dead, of course, but you get the idea. I was smarter than that. I wasn't going to haul around a tattoo by some big-name artist just because of glitter appeal. There needed to be more. I wanted it to empower me. If all I wanted was a decoration, I'd buy a hat.

I had to find the consummate artist. Someone who would be part of my left arm for the rest of my life. A man with machismo. A power figure capable of knocking the block off anyone who threatened me. Someone who, just by putting on the tattoo, would transfer his energy, his life force, his strength of spirit into my bloodstream. Someone whose *mana* would forever be infused in mine.

That person is Bob Roberts.

MIND GAMES

I chose Bob for several reasons. First, he scares the shit out of me. Here's the way I figure it: If Bob Roberts does my tattoo, we'll have a special bond. One of his tattoos makes us almost family, right? I'm not saying Bob Roberts is a bad person. Hey, they used to call him "Buffalo" Bob, and he played saxophone with Ruben and the Jets. It's just that Bob upends my rhythm. I ask him a question, and he'll just stare at me. Like he's sizing me up. It makes me nervous. I function best with lots of feedback. A cheery smile. A nod of the head. A giggle. Bob doesn't do any of that shit. It puts me in a cold sweat when he does that silent thing. I come unglued: *Is he studying that mole on my face? Is he thinking what a jerk I am to have a mole on my face? Does he know I have trouble shaving around it every morning? Does he see that little patch of stubble?*

My guess is that Bob is coming down from a creative high. When I'm writing and someone comes into my office, it takes me a few seconds to adjust, to come back down to Earth. I'm careful not to operate heavy machinery. Maybe it's the same with Bob Roberts. Maybe he's coming back to reality, shifting gears before he talks to writers with moles. I work best when people respond. I don't do well with people who, when you ask them a question, look you right in the eye and say nothing. Maybe Bob is just being honest. He's not interested in pussyfooting around. When he's quiet, he's quiet. But when he gets started, he takes no prisoners.

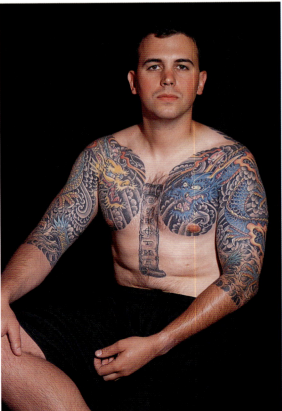

Communication is not his problem. My lord, Bob Roberts is one of the most interesting, articulate men I've ever met. Once he gets rolling, you have to take notes. He's a wealth of information, double entendres, racy stories, and history lessons—enough to choke a college professor. It's his aura that's unnerving. It's his ambiance. His pedigree. He worked side by side with Cliff Raven and Don Ed Hardy, for heaven's sake. Plus a stint with Colonel Todd at the Pike. If that isn't enough, Bob was the man to take over Bert Grimm's chair when Bert left Orange County. No two ways about it, Bob Roberts is the real deal.

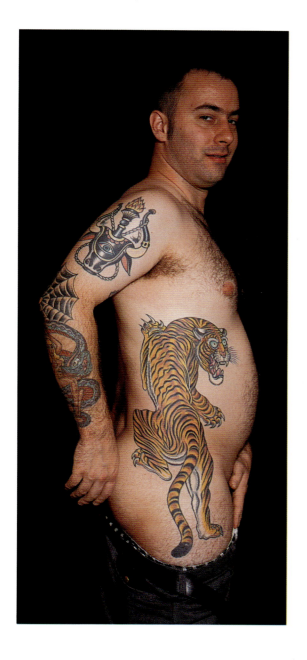

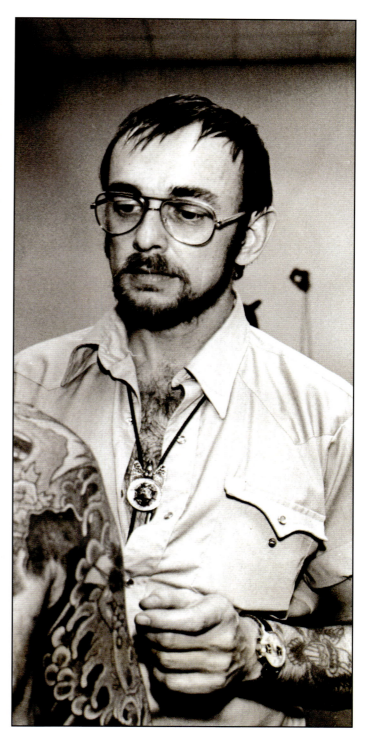

Cliff Raven, Los Angeles, California, 1970s. *Photo courtesy of Tattoo Archive.*

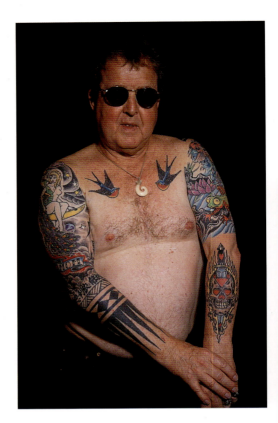

So, when people see my tattooed forearm and ask who did it, I say, "Bob Roberts. You got a problem with that?"

Bob Roberts is the best. I told him I wanted a skull with a banner that said LOVE HURTS. Bob said, "No. Instead of words, I'll say 'love hurts' with the tattoo." And that he did. Up one side and down the other, he drew a skull and dagger, surrounded by flames. And, to mark my past, five broken hearts. The point of the dagger points outward, protecting me.

So far, so good.

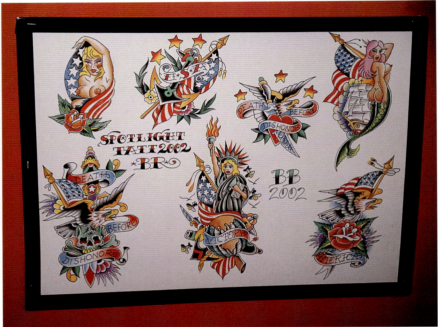

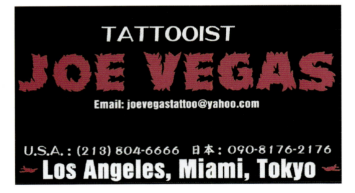

BRYAN BURK AND JOE VEGAS

When Suzanne and I arrived at Spotlight, the usual gang was there: Bob, of course, Bryan Burk, Dennis DeGuzman, and Charlie, Bob's son. Halfway through the shoot, my old pal Joe Vegas showed up with his living canvasses. Joe grew up with my sons Jesse and Riley in Las Vegas. Joe was a big help when I first started editing SKIN & INK. Back then, in the '90s, he worked with my boys at Body Electric. For the last couple years, Joe's been on the road, from Pasadena to Miami. Now he's back in L.A. I hadn't seen any of his handiwork for a while, but, I must say, Joe, as well as everyone in Bob's shop, is committed to the Spotlight legend. But then, I don't think Bob Roberts would put up with inferior work.

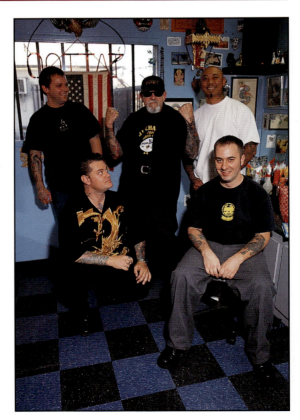

(l. to r.) The shop dogs, Charlie, Joe, Bob, Juan, and Bryan.

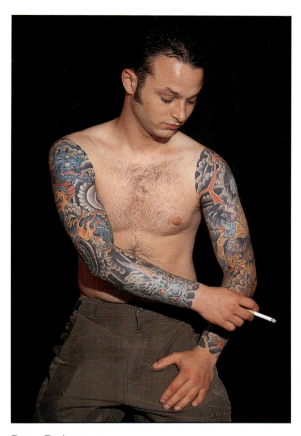

Bryan Burke tattoo.

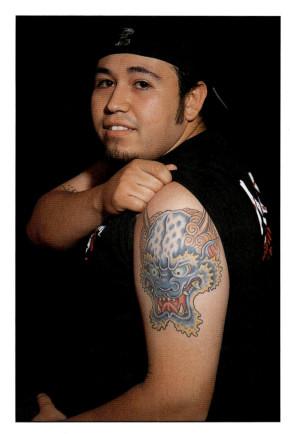

Bryan Burke Tattoo.

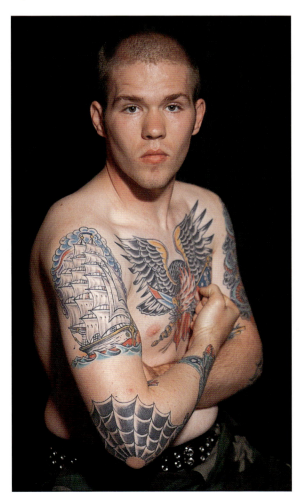

Bryan Burke Tattoo.

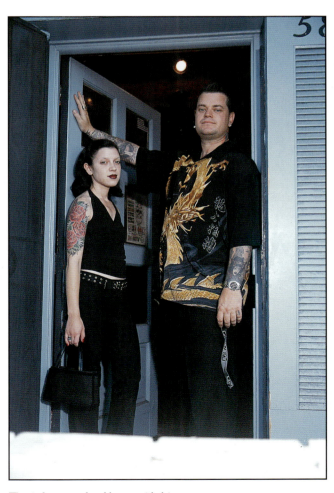

The infamous Joe Vegas with his canvas.

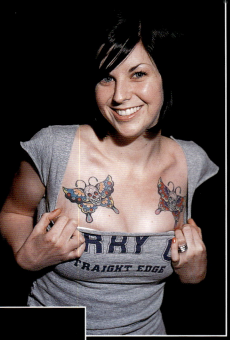

Joe Vegas Tattoos.

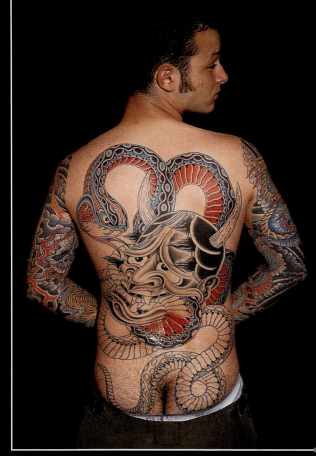

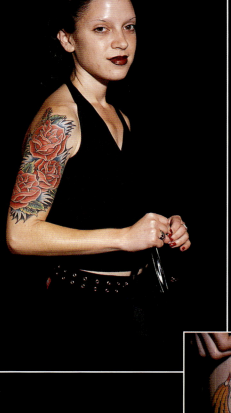

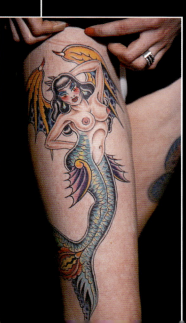

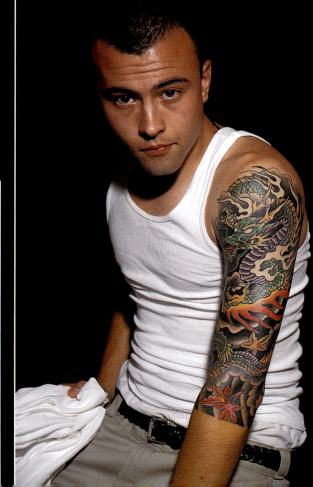

COVERED WITH GREASE

While we were waiting for people to arrive, Baby Ray called to say he was stuck under a car and couldn't make it. "Because of the grease, I look like a living tribal tattoo," he said. "I'll catch you later." Bummer. I definitely wanted to include Ray, but, nevertheless, the shop was percolating. Lots of chitchat, cigarette smoke and Bob expounding on the sorry state of the art world. Yet through all the smoke and monologues, the main thing was the excitement in Bob's voice when he talked about his paintings. He brought out some color prints. He turned the pages and explained each subtle detail. But he wouldn't let me borrow any photos. "They've been published before," he said. "I'll get you new ones."

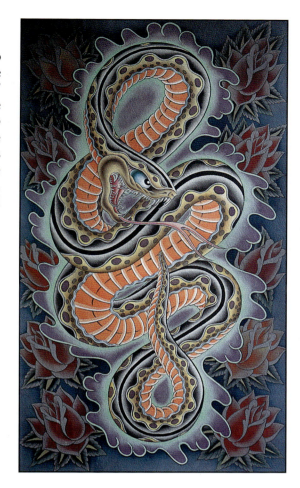

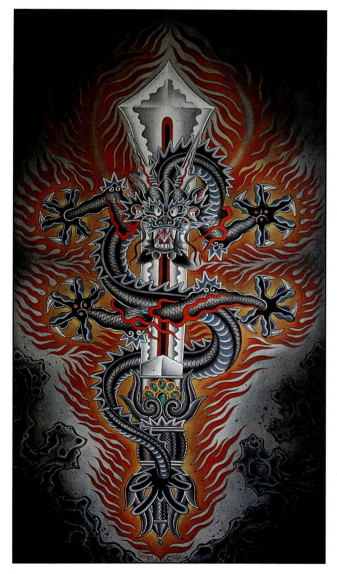

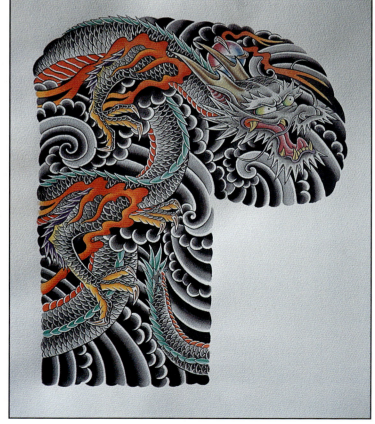

Bob's new graphic work.

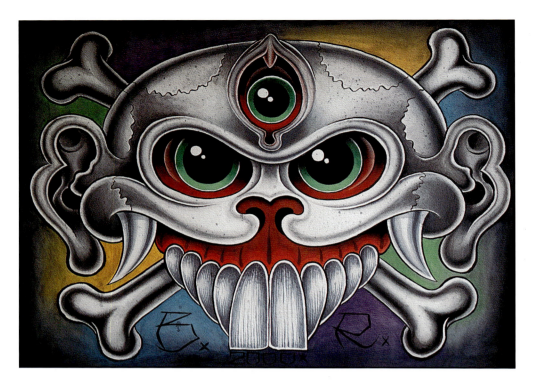

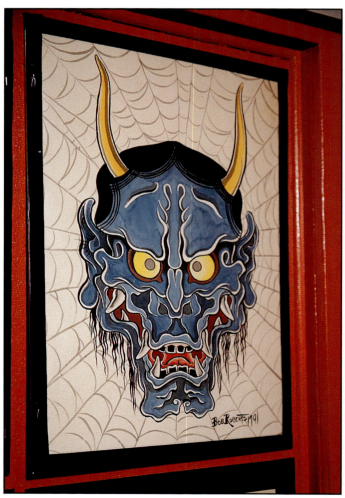

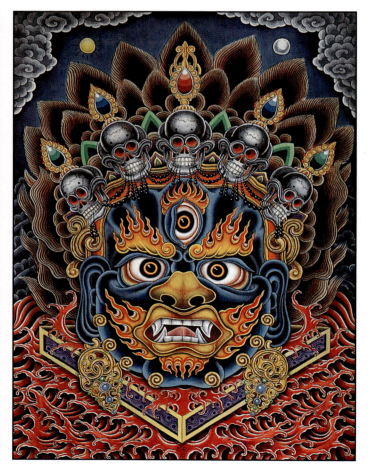

More of Bob's graphic work.

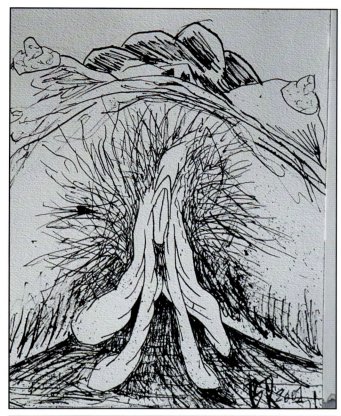

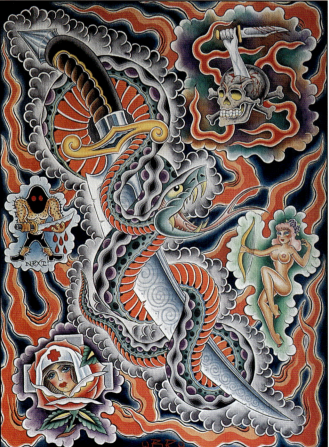

As usual, visiting Spotlight was memorable. A pilgrimage to L.A.'s triple-A power shop. Yes, Bob Roberts is intimidating. Sure, he doesn't pull his punches. Yes, it's humbling to enter his domain, and rightly so. So much of the mystery, the magic, the awe has disappeared from modern-day tattooing. Most of the hard-nosed, motherfucker tattoo shops have been replaced by tattoo salons and poser parlors. But Bob Roberts harkens back to the good old days, when hanging out was a rush and ink on your arms scared people. Spotlight Tattoo is a no-bullshit boutique. Thank God for that. Thank God there's one great, kick-ass shop still left. One smoke-filled, hard-boiled altar where you can get a tattoo that actually looks like a fuckin' tattoo. I'm proud to know Bob Roberts, and I'm proud to wear his skull and dagger on my arm.

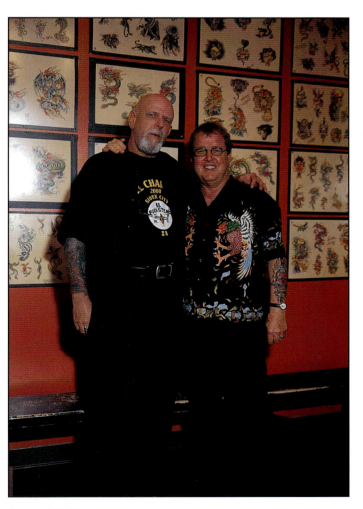

Bob and Bob.

PAT FISH
TATTOO SANTA BARBARA,
SANTA BARBARA, CALIFORNIA

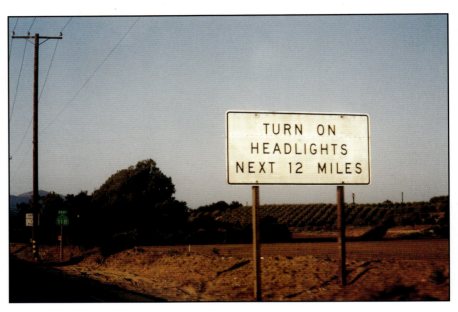

Turn On Headlights Next 12 Miles. What a pleasure to see that sign. It meant I was on a back road. A back road to Santa Barbara, to be exact. The people who put up those signs know, headlights reduce head-ons. When some idiot in a shiny BMW is hurtling toward you at 80 mph crosses the line to pass a truck full of tomatoes, with their headlights blazing, you can see 'em coming. Sure, the six-lane freeway is safer and more time-efficient, but you can't beat zipping down a single-lane blacktop with nothing up ahead but smashed bugs on the windshield. Yeah, momma! For those with the adventuring spirit, California is back-road heaven.

Another benefit is the scenery. Quaint little farmhouses. Rusty old tractors. Sleepy milk cows. Lemon groves and strawberries. When I was a kid, the only way you got anywhere was back roads. And every so often was an oasis—those big, concrete juice stands in the shape of an orange. There you were, hot air blasting through the wind wings, outside like a blast furnace, steam whistling from the radiator, and up ahead—only a mile or two further—ice-cold orange juice. Heaven. It's another unforgettable landmark Southern California will never see again.

One of the last remaining outposts from those glory days is the fruit and vegetable stand. A few miles west of Fillmore is an especially nice one. Peterson Farms Produce. I stopped to take a picture of the avocados and met Laura; Laura and her magnificent fingernails.

"They took three years to grow," she told me.

C'mon, you ain't gonna see that if you take the freeway!

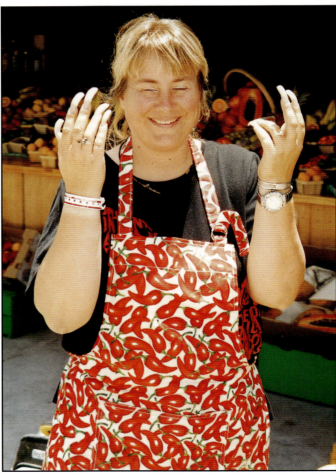

Laura and her splendiferous fingernails.

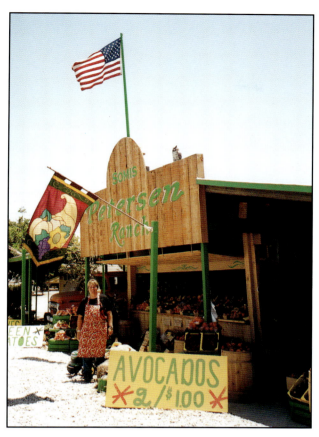

Petersen Ranch produce stand.

TIME TO REFLECT

It's best to focus on the smaller pleasures. In California, trying to capture the enormity, the expanse, all 360 degrees, everything all at once—it's almost impossible. California is simply too big for the camera lens. Like the ride up the 101: The ocean spreads out like a throbbing, blue-green carpet on one side of the road, the rolling, sun-baked, wheat-colored hills on the other. It's beyond description. You need to be there.

Just a few miles north of the 118 cutoff, I spotted another remnant of the old days: a weather-beaten El Camino Real road-sign bell. When I was a kid, I used to count them, those tarnished reminders that 101 was once a cattle trail. Father Junipero Serra, the Spanish priest, established nine Franciscan missions along this road in the late-1700s. His Santa Barbara Mission, state historical landmark #309, founded December 4, 1786, is well worth seeing—if you like missions, that is.

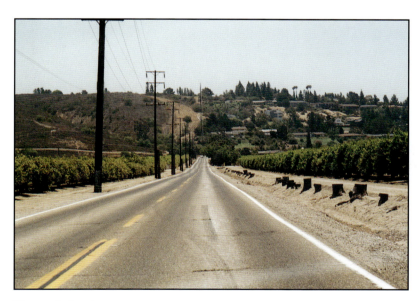

The road ahead.

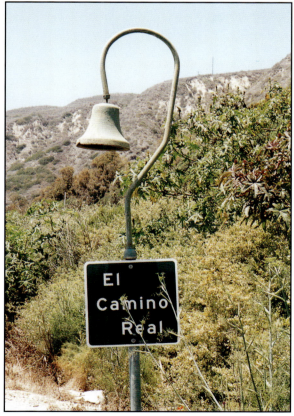

If my memory serves me, the mission bell sounds like someone clanging two garbage cans together. But it doesn't make any difference. There was a parade right up the middle of State Street, and I couldn't get to Mission Avenue. But the big deal isn't the mission anyway, it's State Street: block after block of boutiques, antiques, restaurants by the score, all within the context of charming, early-California architecture. And after you window shop for a couple hours, there's an amazing pier built over the ocean, a great view of the yacht harbor and, on weekends, sidewalk art shows. But that's not why I traveled 114 miles. I was there to visit the "Queen of Celt." The inimitable Pat Fish.

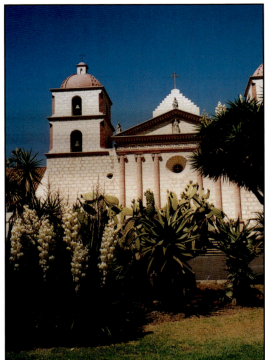

Mission Santa Barbara (I went back a month later and got the shot).

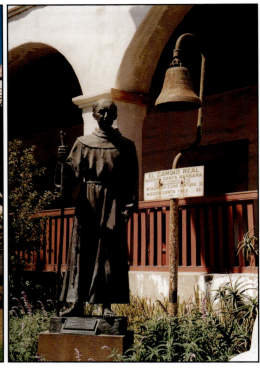

Father Serra with his bell.

THE ONE, THE ONLY

Everyone knows Pat Fish. A local since 1975, Pat put herself through college, receiving degrees in both art and film from the University of California in Santa Barbara. Following that, Pat was a reporter for the local newspaper and a professor of art at the community college. In 1984, Pat decided to become a full-time tattoo artist, learning the fine points from the late Cliff Raven, just before Cliff decided to sell Sunset Strip Tattoo and open Raven's Bookshop in 29 Palms. This is good, and this is bad. Good because people travel from the far corners of the universe for an official Pat Fish Celtic tattoo. Bad because of the negative reaction to many of her comments on the current tattoo scene. Add to this the fact that besides virtually cornering the tattoo market in this one of the most wonderful towns on the planet, Pat's beautifully designed Web site, www.luckyfish.com, gets about 80 zillion hits a day. Could there possibly be a touch of resentment that Ms. Fish is also a savvy businesswoman and successful entrepreneur in an industry dominated by men?

Naaah.

All this aside, I received a warm welcome from the Queen and was promptly escorted into her library by two enthusiastic handmaidens. I was a bit disappointed that Pat's 180-pound Irish wolfhound, Nemo, wasn't there, but there were plenty of tropical fish and people to look at. It was especially nice to see Pat's workmate, Paul Votava, an old friend of Joe Vegas.

Click-click, pop-pop—the photography went pretty smoothly, and my stomach was growling. Due to the cordoned-off streets and me missing the new off-ramp, I was behind schedule and about to faint from malnutrition. La Super-Rica!

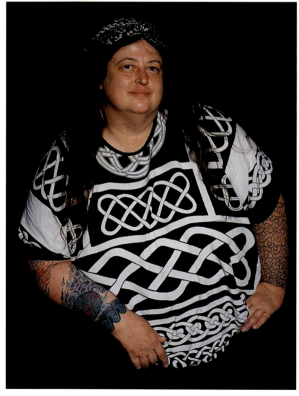

The famous one, Pat Fish.

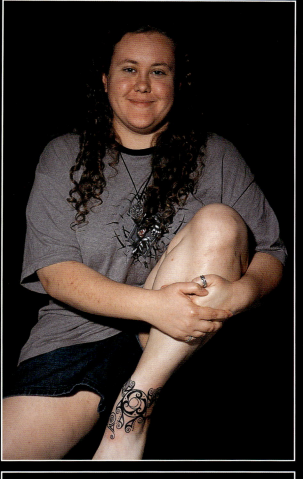
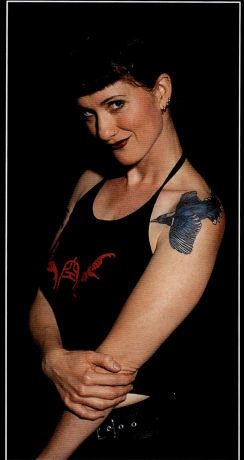
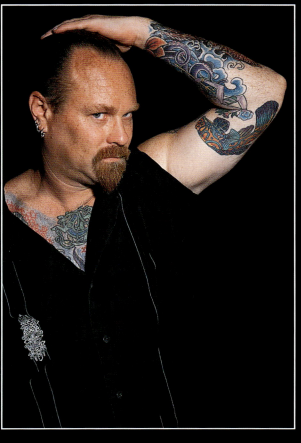
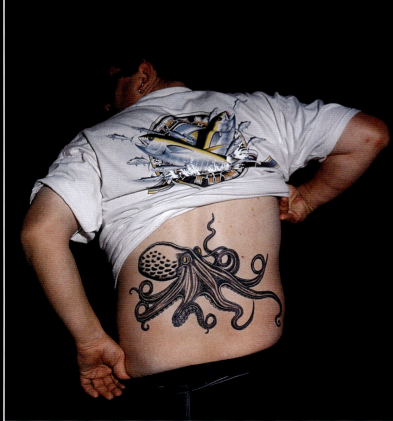

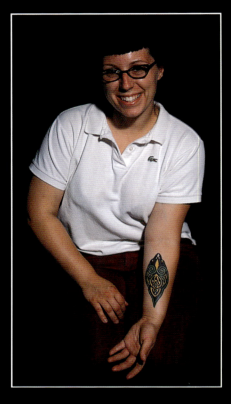
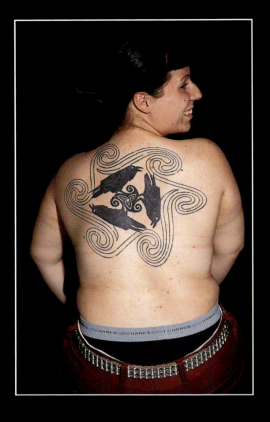
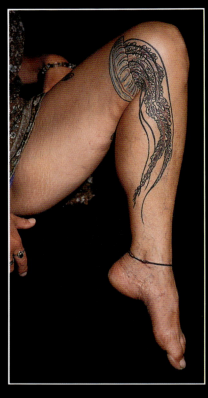
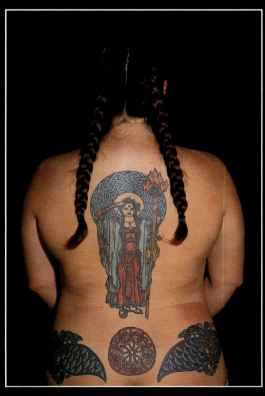
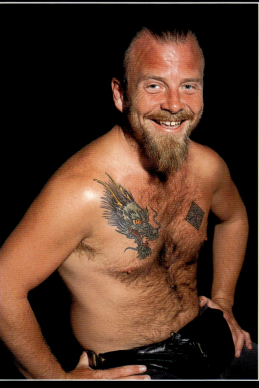
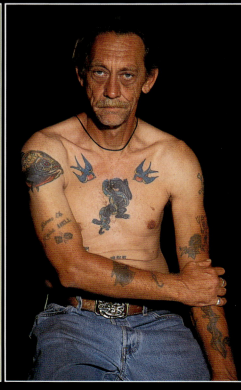

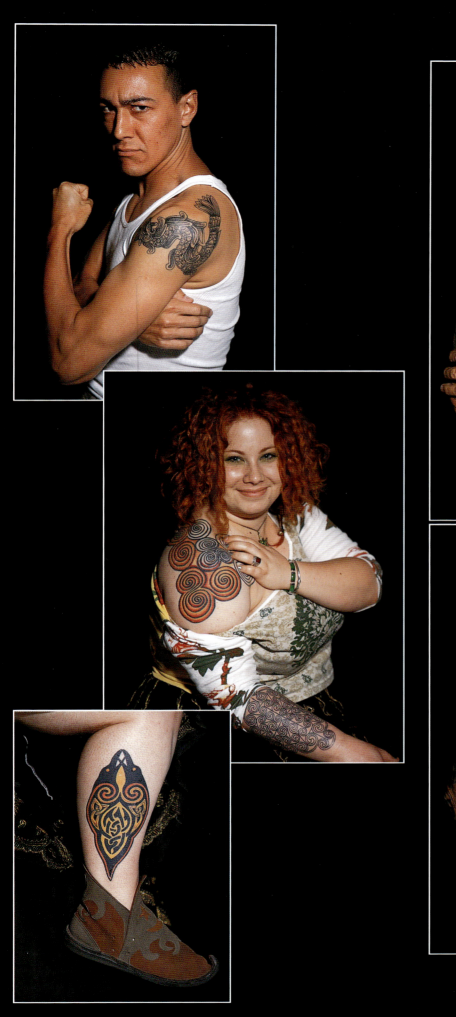
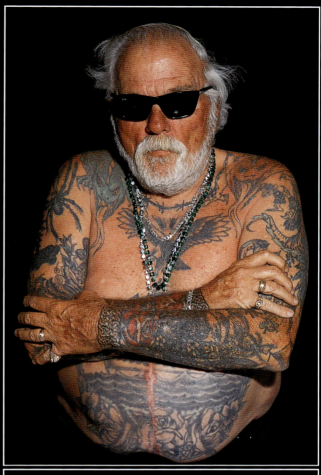
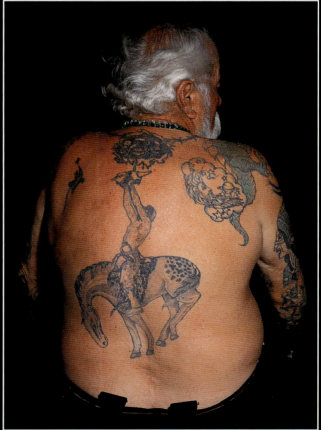

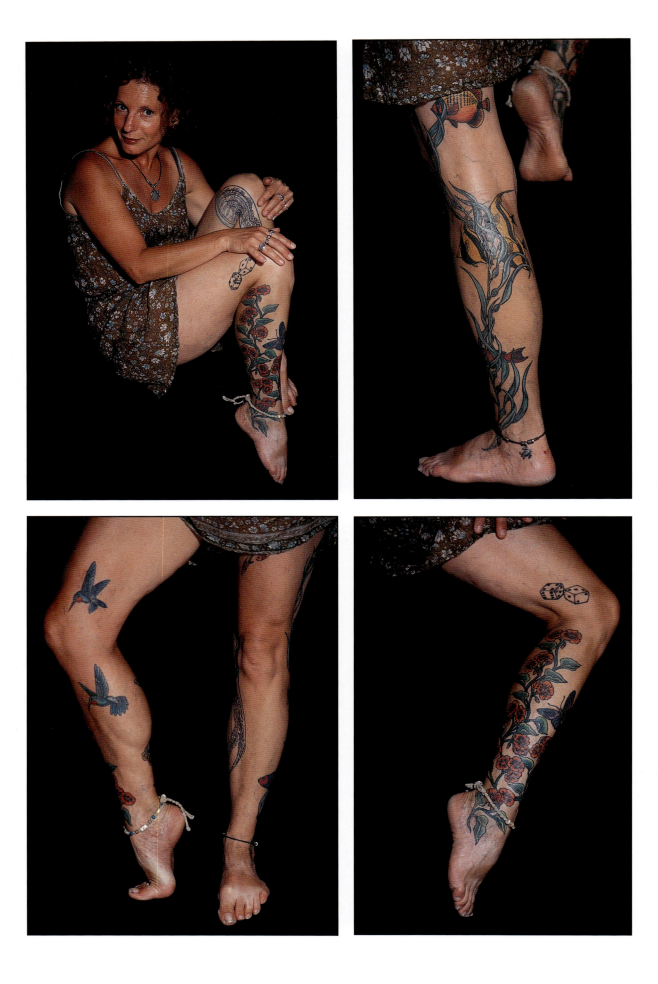

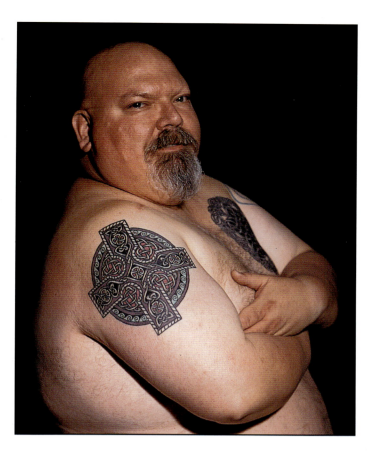

COMIDA TIME

I love La Super-Rica Taqueria. An unassuming corner building with no visible sign outside (you can spot it by the crowd out front), La Super-Rica makes super-good Mexican food. Here's the deal: You wait in line, scan the menu on the wall and order from the hombre at the counter. Parked at the edge of a residential neighborhood, La Super-Rica got famous when Julia Child sampled the fare a few years back. Obviously, eating unpretentious food off a paper plate with a plastic fork and sitting in a vine-covered patio on plastic chairs did not diminish the enthusiasm of either Ms. Child or myself for this, the sine qua non of Southern California Mexican cuisine.

I love visiting Pat Fish.

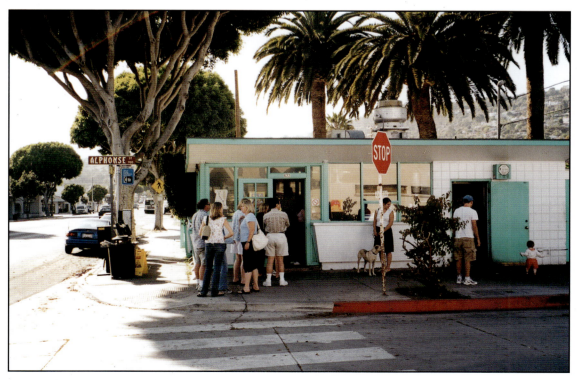

Yum! La Super Rica.

JACK RUDY
GOOD TIME CHARLIE'S
TATTOOLAND, ANAHEIM

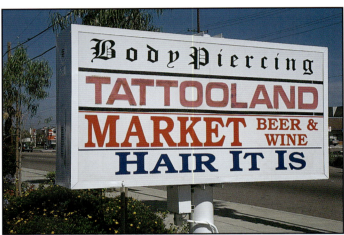

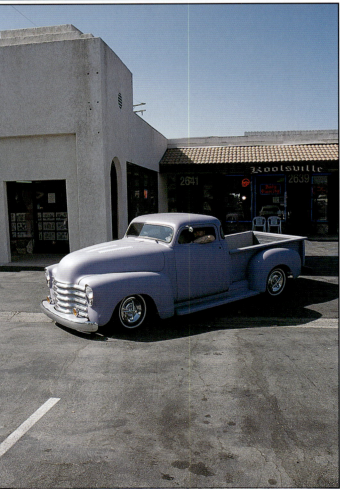

I made an appointment with Jack for three o'clock. I took it as a compliment when this kingpin of 21st century tattooing pulled up a mere quarter of an hour late in his purple pickup with the Frenched taillights.

"Man, I can't believe I'm 15 minutes late," said Jack, as he climbed out of the cab. "I'm never that on time."

A tough-looking guy in a tough-looking car, Jack Rudy was born in downtown Los Angeles. When Jack was a kid, his parents took him to the Pike, and when he was six, Jack watched the sailors coming out of Bert Grimm's. They'd say stuff like, "Hey, man, my tattoo's better than yours." And the other guy would say, "Fuck you, mine's better."

Wow, thought little Jack. *I want a tattoo!*

"I never dreamed I'd be putting them on," he remembers. "I did my first one by hand when I was 15 and started making homemade machines when I was 17. When I was 19, home from Marine Corps boot camp, I met Good Time Charlie Cartwright. A friend of mine wanted me to tattoo him, but my machine was running half-assed. I didn't exactly know what was wrong with it, much less fuck around with it. So I said, 'Let's go down to the Pike and see if anyone's good down there.' I wanted to go there anyway, before they closed it down. It was in 1974."

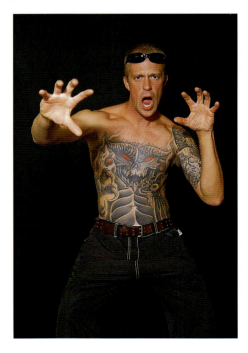

Jack arrives in style.

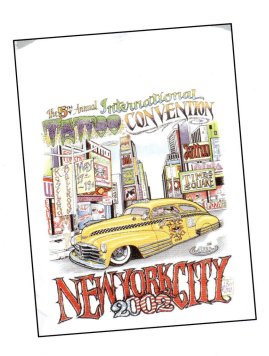

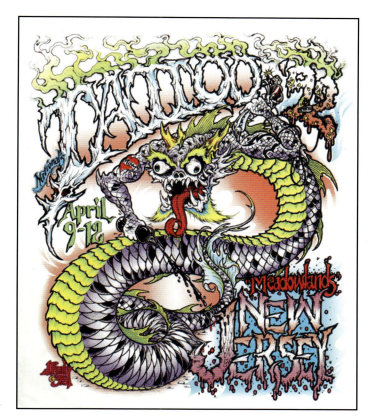

A VISIT TO THE PIKE

"We went into Bert Grimm's first, but that was too crowded. Then we went to Lee Roy's next door. They still had flash up on the walls from World War II. That wouldn't do, so we tried the next one. And the next. Then we got to the end. The Rose, it was called. A bar converted into a tattoo shop. That's where I met Good Time Charlie. He tattooed my friend. I went back a couple times. Charlie and I became friends. I liked Charlie. I hung out over the next year and a half.

"I remember asking if he could set me up with some machines, not knowing, of course, that a machine was just the beginning. But Charlie said, 'Yeah, I'll fix you up.' What I didn't realize was, Charlie was going to apprentice me. When I heard that, I was thrilled. Good Time Charlie was going to teach me the business! So, when I got out of the Marine Corps in '75, I went to work with him. He was leaving the Pike, and I said, 'Charlie, I know a really great place to open a tattoo shop.' He said, 'Where?' And I said, 'East L.A., man. That would be a really cool place.' Charlie said, 'You know what? I've been thinking the same thing.' And so he opened up on Whittier Boulevard. He called me that summer, after I got out, and I started working for him. It was called Good Time Charlie's Tattoo Parlor.

"I was fresh out of the Corps. In fact, I was tattooing before I had a professional tattoo myself. People would come into the shop—I had real short hair and couldn't even grow a moustache. They'd look at Charlie, and they'd look at me and say, 'If it's all right with you, homes, I'm just gonna wait for Charlie.' I looked like the amateur I was. Charlie had long hair, a cool biker-looking dude. Hey, I didn't even look my age.

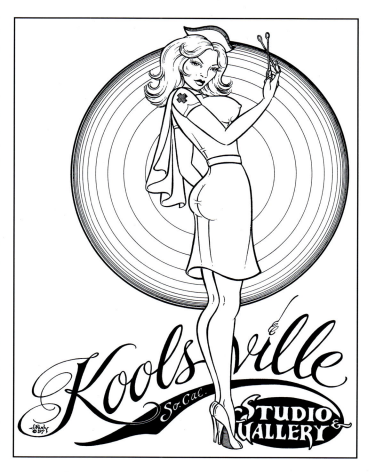

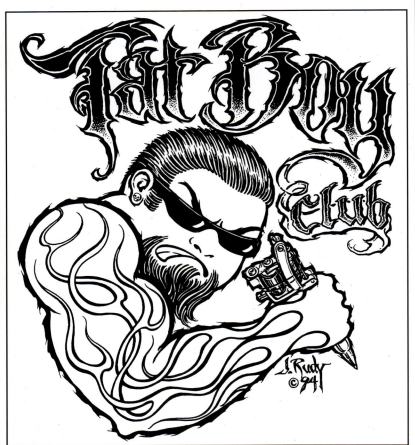

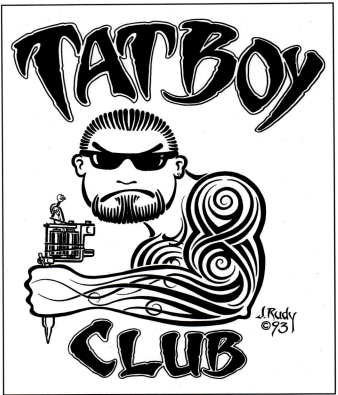

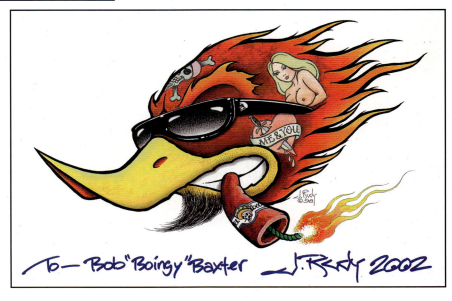

To—Bob "Boingy" Baxter   J. Rudy 2002

"Charlie and I started doing single-needle work at the same time. We took a three, modified it and came up with a single. We started doing that sometime in '76. We kept at it from then on. So when Charlie and I went to our first convention, Reno in 1977, we met Ed Hardy, Bob Roberts, Mike Malone—guys we'd heard of and were already legendary in the tattoo world, along with legitimate old-timers, of course, like Bob Shaw, Colonel Todd, Paul Rogers. It was quite an experience for us. Reno was the second major tattoo convention ever held in the United States.

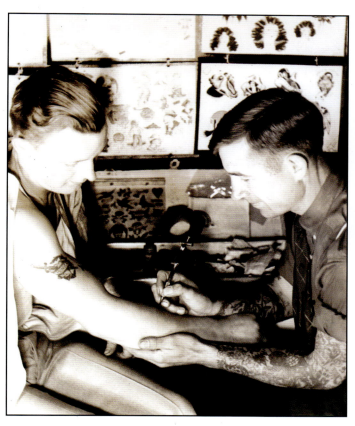

Paul Rogers tattooing in Jacksonville, North Carolina, 1950s.
Photo courtesy of Tattoo Archive.

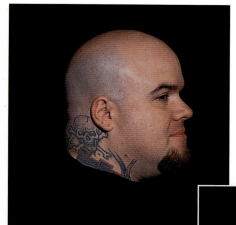

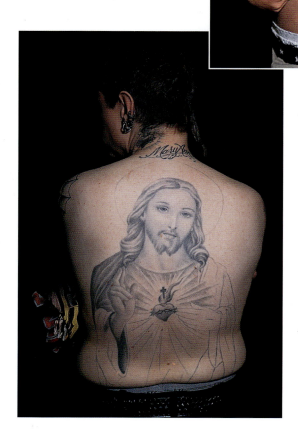

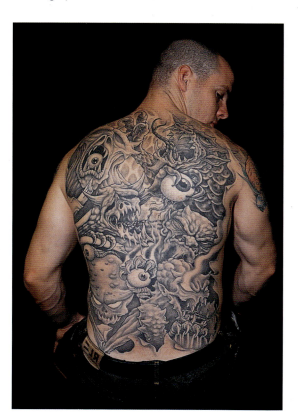

69

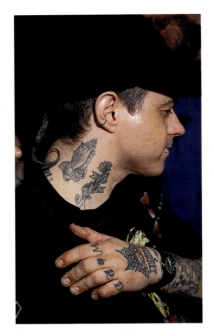

IN AT THE BEGINNING

"The very first convention was in Houston, 1976. We were considering going to that one, but thought, *Tattoo convention? What the hell's that? What are we going to do there? Is that like a plumbers' convention?* Anyway, we didn't go. We thought we'd hear how it was and decide after that. So when they had one in Reno—which was infinitely closer than Texas—we went and had a ball. We took a guy with us that we'd both done a lot of black and gray on. Actually the main reason for going was to meet Ed, Don Ed Hardy. But he always had an entourage. Even in those days. There was a group of people around him, so why would he want to talk to us? The notorious nobodies from East L.A. Maybe we'd get a chance later. Then, somehow, Ed saw the work we did on this guy, and he goes, "Wow, what's going on with this black and gray stuff?" Then he sought *us* out. It was really quite a surprise. We were thinking, *When are we going to get a chance to talk to him?* As busy as the guy is, he comes and finds us! After that, Ed came down with Malone and Bob Roberts to the shop in East L.A.—and everybody got tattooed.

"Sure, Freddy Negrete was doing single-needle nonprofessionally way before me and Charlie, but, as far as a professional shop goes, we started the whole thing. I think George Burchett was doing single-needle tattooing in England. I saw some of his flash from the old days, and I can't imagine doing that stuff except single-needle. I don't know for a fact that anyone was doing it way before we did, but, if that's true, we reinvented it in 1976.

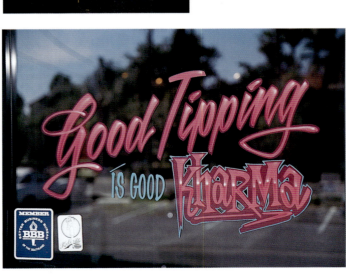

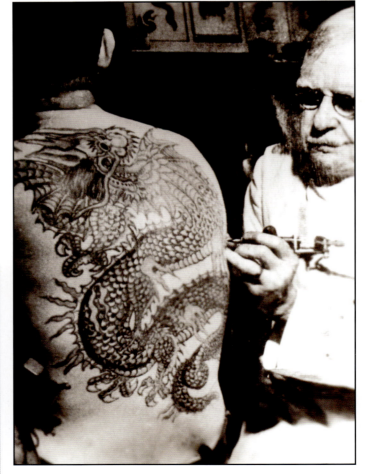

George Burchett tattooing, London, England, 1940s. *Photo courtesy of Tattoo Archive.*

"Charlie lasted in East L.A. for a couple years. Then he moved to Kansas and sold the business to Ed Hardy. This was 1977 or '78. At that time it was just me and Freddy Negrete. I stayed in East L.A. on Whittier Boulevard for nine and a half years. Freddy got religion in 1980 and quit tattooing altogether. By the time 1984 came around, we closed down the East L.A. shop. Mark Mahoney was working for me at that time. Flame McNorton, he worked for me a couple years. And the notorious Mike Brown and his Band of Renown. Even Kate Hellenbrand worked there. In 1984, they sold the property, but there was no way I could afford it, so I moved to Anaheim. I've been here for the last 17 years. It was the fourth shop in all of Orange County. I think little Dave Spellman had one in Santa Ana. Patty Pavlik had one in Newport Beach. There was Twilight Fantasy and another one, Anaheim Tattoo. But they went out of business shortly before I arrived. There was only a handful of shops in Orange County. Those were the days."

I like talking to Jack. There are very few people as honest. When you talk with Jack Rudy, you don't just listen, you learn. You learn the difference between second string and the real deal. You learn that there's too many goddam tattoo shops. You learn that starter kits are crap. You learn about a flurry of stupid things members of the tattoo community have done in the name of arrogance and money.

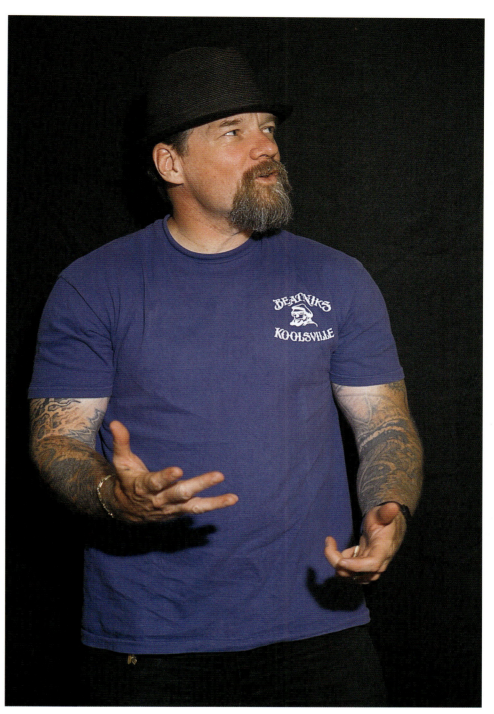

Jack.

Sure, you can disagree with Jack Rudy. But it won't do you any good. He's too smart, and he's too experienced. He's contributed way too much to be disregarded, and he's too hard-nosed to push around. With the advent of tattoo shops on every corner and self-proclaimed "arteests" patrolling the aisles of far too many conventions, there are few unimpeachable icons like Jack. I'm proud to say he's a friend. A supporter of just causes. A legend in his own time. And, to many of us, the essence of what tattooing is all about. But above all, he'll always be Jack Fuckin' Rudy.

VISIT 8
JUDY PARKER
PACIFIC TATTOOS, SAN DIEGO

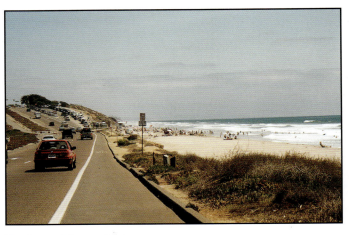
The beautiful coast highway.

I looked forward to spending some time with Judy Parker—even though it meant another long drive to San Diego. Our meeting was set for 8 p.m. That meant, if I left at five, I'd glide up to her door with time to spare. Except on Friday, with all that bumper-to-bumper traffic. *Hmmmmm. What if I left directly from my 11 a.m. cover meeting at Larry Flynt's, got on the road by noon and beat the crush? There'd be plenty of time for a leisurely luncheon.*

Well, so much for that. The interstate was a parking lot. It was stop start, stop start, stop start all the way to Irvine. I might not have left early enough.

I decided to take Highway 1, the two-lane route that hugs the coastline. There are stoplights, but it's way prettier than the 5. I exited at Oceanside. The scenery improved almost immediately. I'm not saying the best route from Pasadena to San Diego is surface streets, but driving 35 mph through Carlsbad, Encinitas, Solana Beach and Del Mar is what California living is all about. Beautiful homes, expansive beaches, suntanned bodies and plenty of freshly waxed surfboards. In fact, two blocks into Oceanside, I spotted cool murals, a fabulous moviehouse marquee and a gorgeous local honey eating fish tacos. There's so much more to see off the freeway.

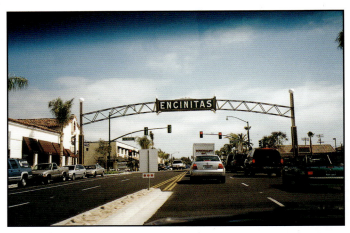

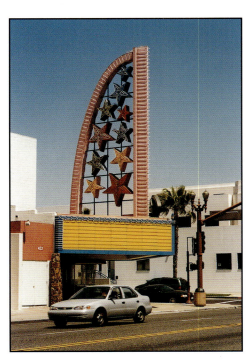

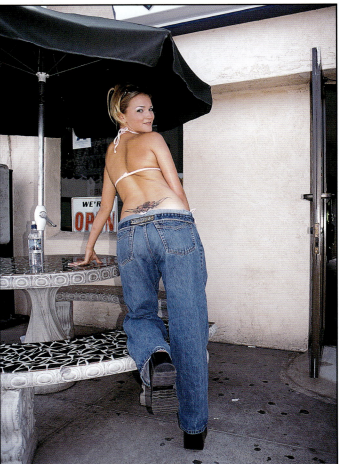
The honey at the taco place.

But the best part was taking pictures from the lifeguard tower. In order to weasel my way up the ladder, I waved a copy of SKIN & INK. "I'm the editor," I told the guard. "Come on up," he said. I flashed a smile, climbed up and joined him at the rail. I handed over the latest issue, the one with an Aaron Bell pinup on the cover. He checked it out, while I scanned the beach through my viewfinder. Perfect weather, perfect surf, gorgeous sun-kissed girls in string bikinis. This was clearly the best possible way for a young man to spend a summer. "What a great job," I said.

"Yes," said the lifeguard, as he flipped through the pages. "I'm really jealous."

I didn't stop to explain I was talking about *him*, but it didn't make any difference. His comment made my day.

A few miles south, the traffic turned hideous—carnival time at the Del Mar Racetrack—so, back on the interstate. I got to San Diego just in time for commuter gridlock. Thank heaven I was headed into town, against traffic. With almost three hours to spare, I headed for Seaport Village, bought a groovy shirt with tribal-style pineapples, photographed some boats and bought popcorn. A word of warning: Do not, under any circumstances, buy popcorn at Seaport Village. The moment the bleedin' seabirds see you, they attack. I was surrounded by 100 little, black, pecky ones. The ringleader was a big, nasty, gray motherfucker. I dumped the popcorn and ran.

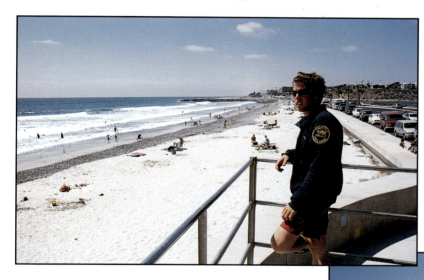

The ever watchful lifeguard.

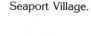

Seaport Village.

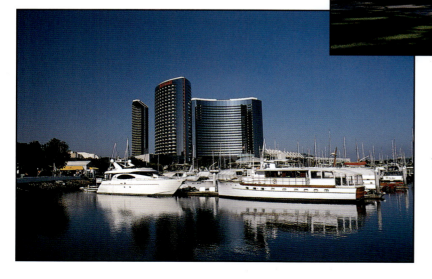

A view of downtown San Diego from Seaport Village.

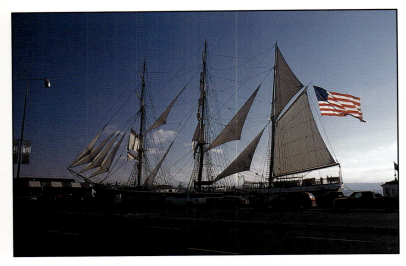

Downtown San Diego isn't too hard to figure out, so I stopped by Dave Gibson's. Dave wasn't there, but Eric the Red was in town doing a guest spot. Luckily, Eric had two Judy Parker tattoos on his arms. Judy said she didn't expect a lot of people at her shoot, so these extras were a nice surprise.

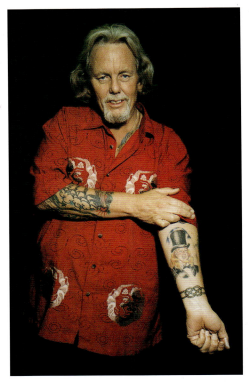

Eric the Red with his Judy Parker artwork.

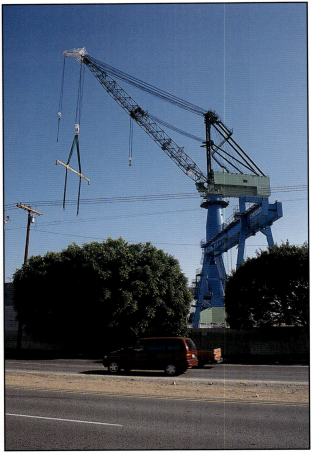

A enormous crane that lifts big, heavy thingies out of humongous cargo vessels.

I got to Pacific Tattoo at sunset. Judy calls it the ghetto. Sure, it's on the wrong side of the tracks and pretty remote, but there's a well-groomed golf course across the street. "It's for the Navy," said Judy. "Every once in a while, a golf ball breaks my windshield. But that's all right, because the military pays for it."

That's good news.

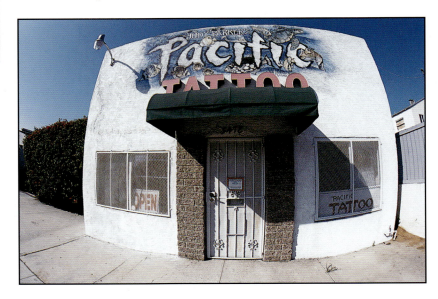

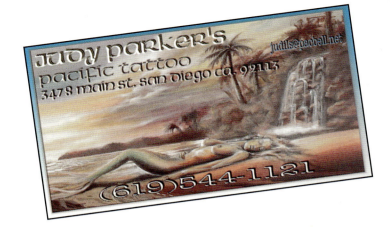

judy parker's
pacific tattoo
3478 main st. san diego ca. 92113
judils@pacbell.net
(619) 544-1121

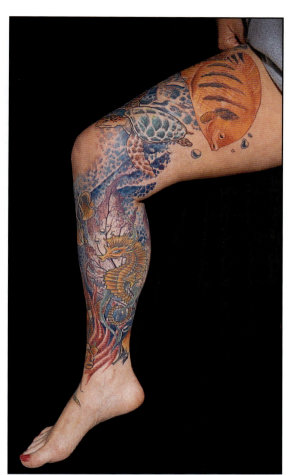

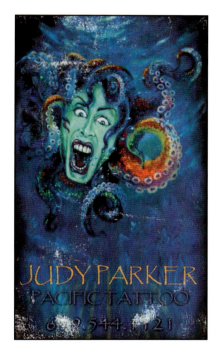

JUDY PARKER
PACIFIC TATTOO
619 544 1121

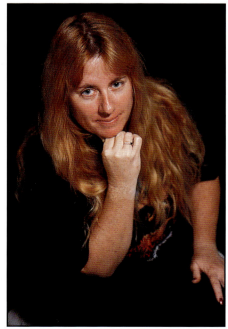

Ms. Judy.

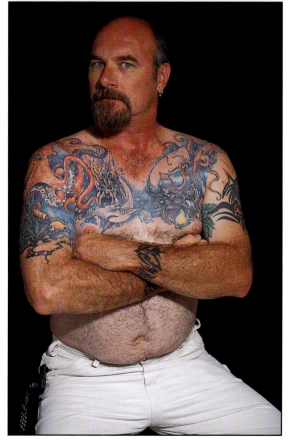

FAMOUS FLASH

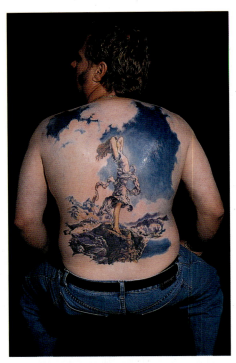

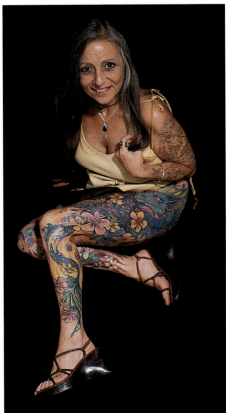

Judy, quiet and girlish, with a mischievous twinkle in her eye, runs a clean, well-organized shop on a street with no foot traffic. Judy keeps her distance from both the center of the San Diego tattoo scene and the neon and lights of mainstream tattooing. The way I heard about Judy Parker was through her flash, and, according to Judy, drawing was a way for her to get her foot in the door.

"Initially, I didn't think my tattoo skills were as high as my art skills, which is why I did a lot of flash. I started getting known because of my flash. I think people took me a lot more seriously than I ever took myself. I never really wanted to tattoo. Steve, a tattoo artist in Alaska, just thrust it into my hand. I had never seen tattooing done before that. I never took it seriously, due to my religious background. And because I didn't take it seriously, I misstepped and missed out on all the training I could have gotten. I didn't think it was a serious career. I was 17 and to me it was a laughed-upon kind of thing. My dad was very, very harsh. He thought of me as the top of not a very good heap. He put tattooing in a very bad light and still does. I'm the black sheep of the family.

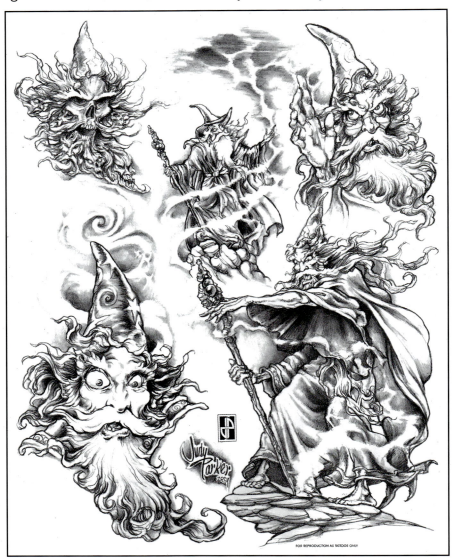

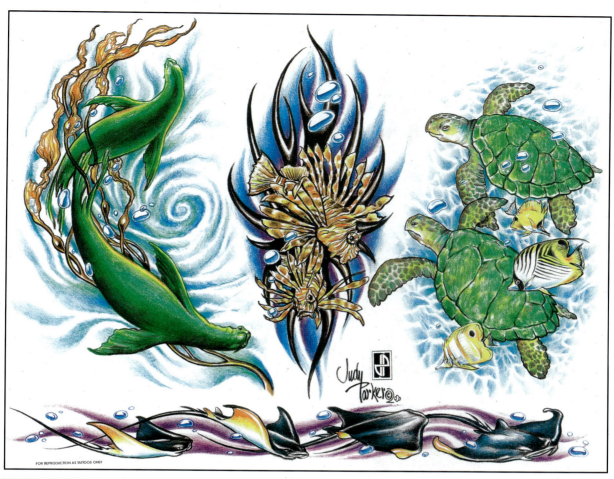

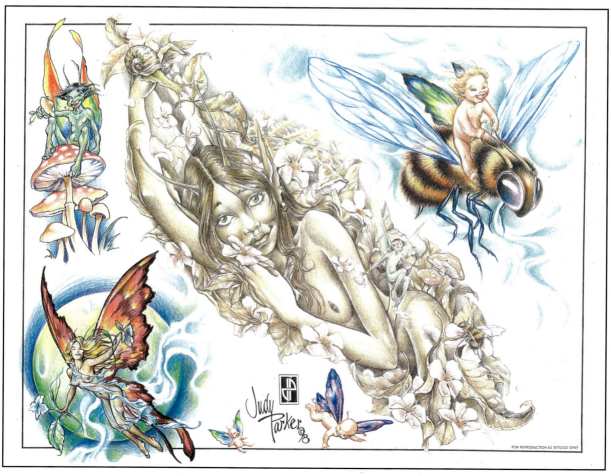

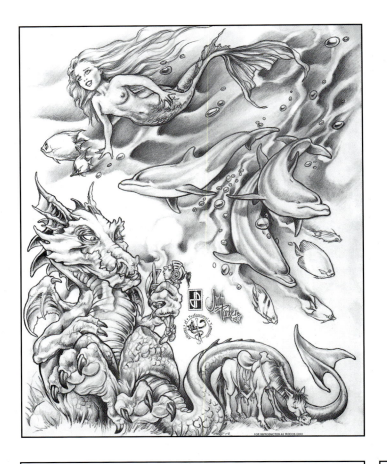

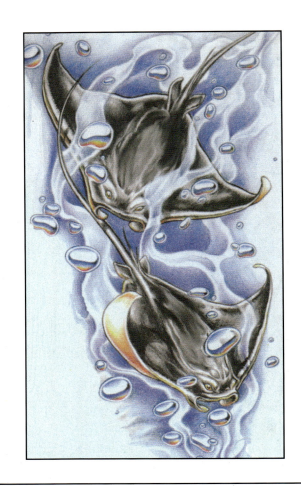

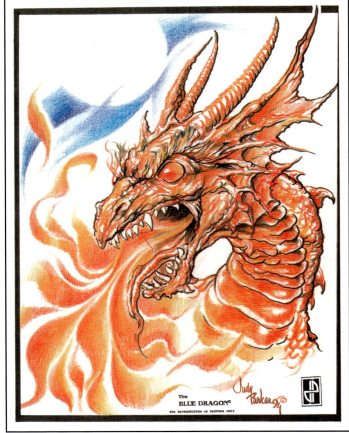

The
BLUE DRAGON

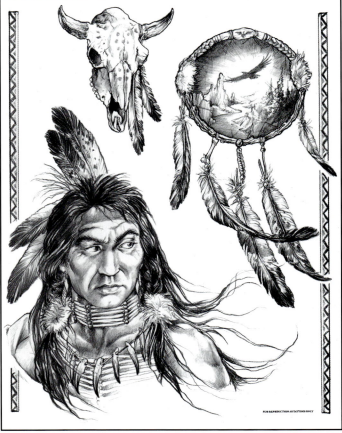

"Consequently, I didn't take tattooing seriously for many years, even when I was working for Doc Webb. I figured I wasn't top dog and didn't consider myself knowledgeable. I started going to conventions in 1990. That's when I finally realized tattooing was important and had value. It wasn't just a carnival-sideshow thing and actually had merit. I didn't get trained until people from conventions began taking me under their wings. People like Sailor Moses and Jack Rudy actually told me how to do it better.

"A lot of people know me because of my flash. I was told to do flash from the beginning. When I worked for Al Orsini in San Diego, I did flash for $5 a day. I had returned to San Diego to be near my mother and go to college to become an art teacher. That didn't work out, so I walked into Doc Webb's and asked him for a job. He was a really nice guy. He treated me really good. That was 1981. I only worked for Doc Webb for a couple years, because Jim Kunkle was getting annoyed. All the sailors were coming to me. They didn't want the guy with the big cigar tattooing them. They wanted the young girl. Then I worked for Al Orsini for a while. He had three shops: Gene's Tattoo Shop, Thunderbolt, and One Stop. Then I opened my first shop, Blue Dragon, in 1984. It was at 31st and Main. Right up the street. I opened my current shop, Judy Parker's Pacific Tattoo, in 1994.

"Through all of this, I got no support from my family. None. The tattoo community has taken over that role—so much so that I feel I could stop anywhere if I had any kind of problems and stay at their homes and be part of their family. I have a very warm feeling for my tattoo family."

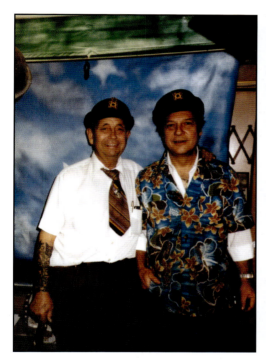

Doc Webb and Trader Jim, San Diego, California, 1960s. *Photo courtesy of Tattoo Archive.*

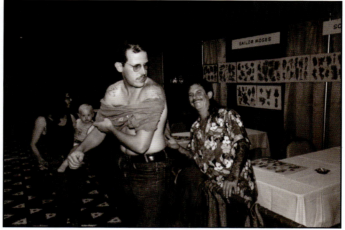

Sailor Moses on the convention floor, 1980s. *Photo courtesy of Tattoo Archive.*

At the Inkslingers Ball, 1993.

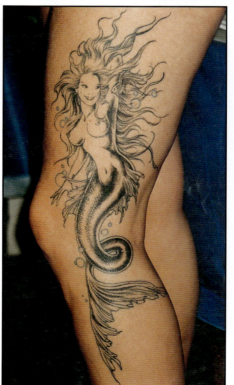

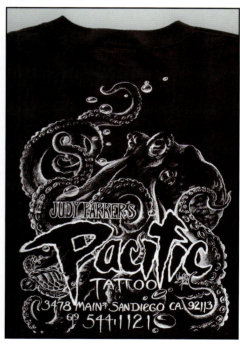

79

BABA AND ODIE
VINTAGE TATTOO, HIGHLAND PARK

Baba learned about the enormous turnout at Mike Pike's shop in Lancaster and vowed to outdo him.

"I take it as a personal challenge," said Baba.

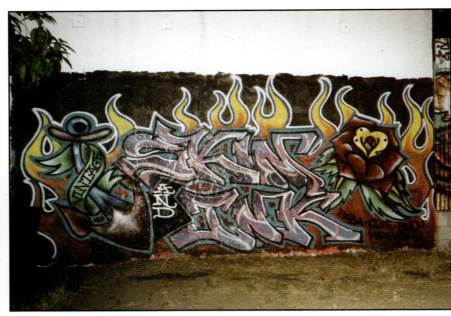

Baba and Odie pay tribute to SKIN & INK.

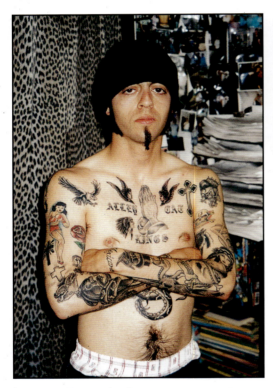

A Vintage Tattoo sampler.

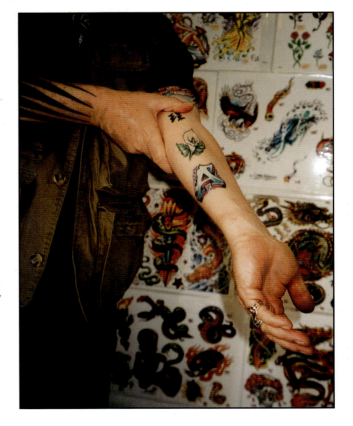

The author's tattoo graffiti A (for grandson Aedan) by Baba.

I'm foggy on the details, but Baba packed the place. Young people, old people, neighbors, strangers—even a big, slobbery bulldog. There were plenty of ice cubes, five kinds of soft drinks, lots of loud music and three pepperoni pizzas. Everybody was bumping everybody. There was no place to sit. There was no place to stand. There wasn't even room for the bulldog! And there I was, camera in hand, getting my toes trampled by the ever-swarming mass of gurgling babies, goateed homeboys, tattooed dudes and lovely ladies.

I prefer privacy, but was forced to set up in the front room. Quite simply, I don't like people looking over my shoulder when I work. Of course, once I started, the wise-ass peanut gallery hooted at anyone I photographed. I'd say to a model, "Pull up your sleeve," and the wolf whistles would start. No time to be self-conscious at Vintage Tattoo. Everyone was on stage. All this, of course, was brilliantly choreographed by the tireless impresario himself, my good friend and protector if I ever get into trouble in a back alley, Baba, the once and forever, un-disputed Tattoo Lord of Highland Park.

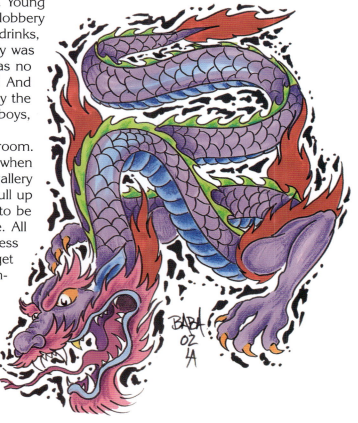

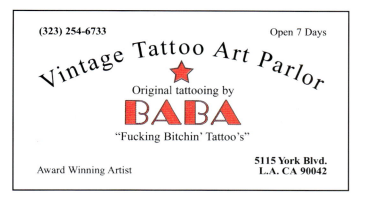

When Baba and his brother Odie were young, they did their art in the dead of night. Instead of applause, the sound they heard was police sirens. Thanks to fast feet and the grace of God, these midnight marauders escaped over the fence with their spray cans. But times change. The boys decided to stop running and start making money. Baba hit the celebrity road, airbrushing stage outfits for Vanilla Ice and his entourage. Lest those halcyon days be forgotten, under Vintage's counter is an armload of scrapbooks and fan magazines featuring the Hot Shit Kid himself, Baba at 22.

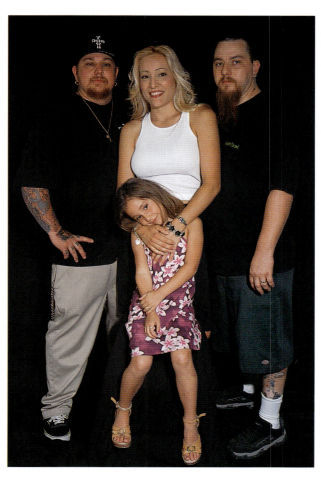

Baba (l.) and Odie, with Baba's wife Kim and daughter, Sierra.

Looking for a more permanent gig, Baba landed in New York City. After figuring out who's who, Baba found Jonathan Shaw through the Yellow Pages. When he asked for a job, Shaw said no. It was 1989, tattooing was illegal in New York, and Shaw worked underground. "Nobody's apprenticing but my wife," said Shaw. But he did invite Baba to watch him work—Sundays, from midnight to five in the morning.

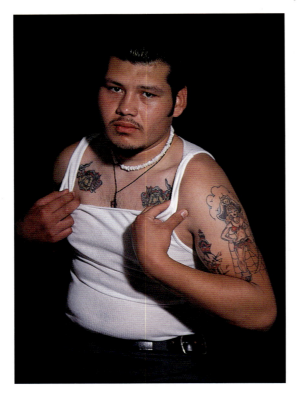
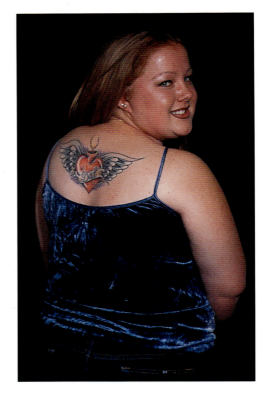

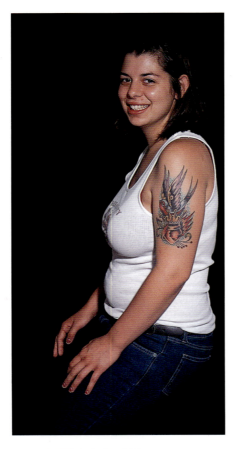
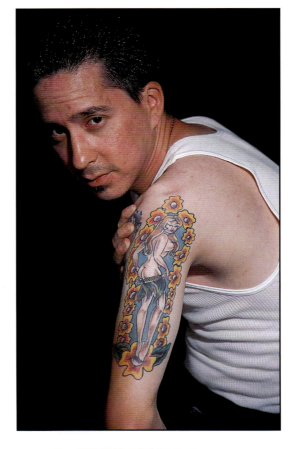

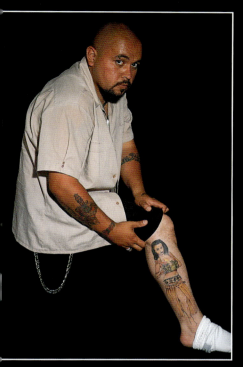

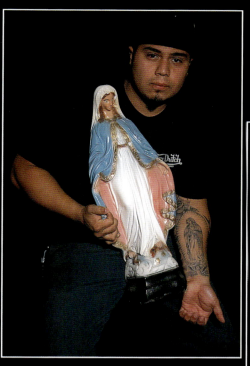

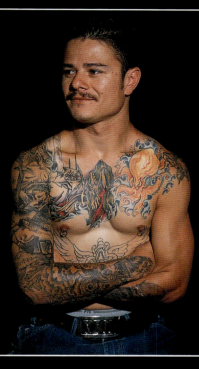

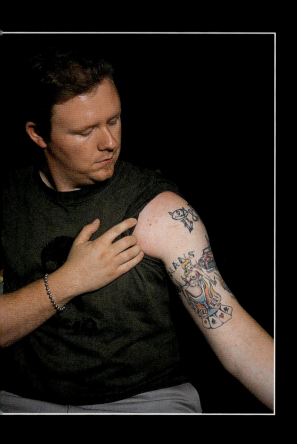

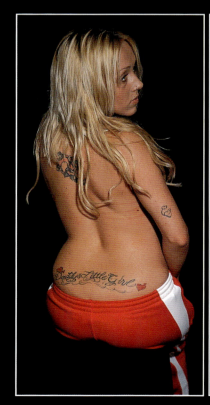

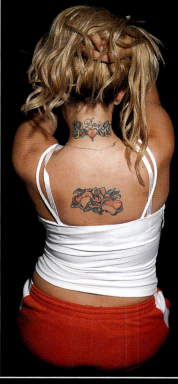

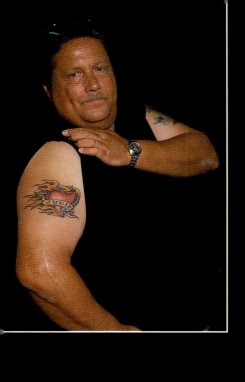
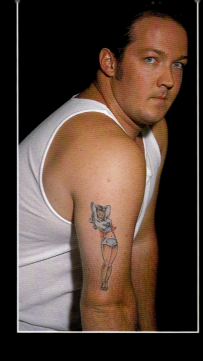
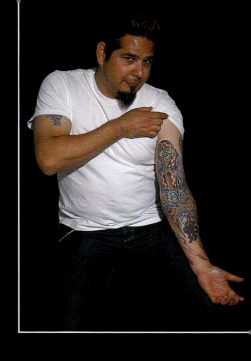
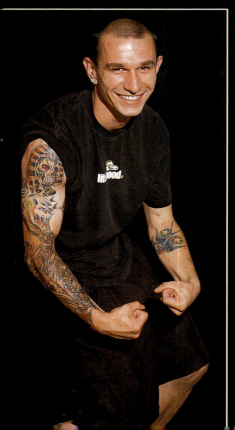
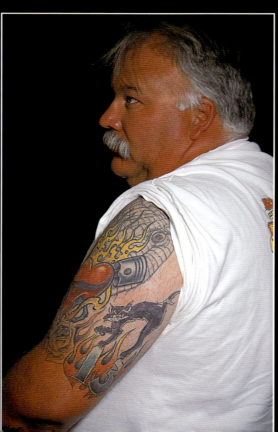
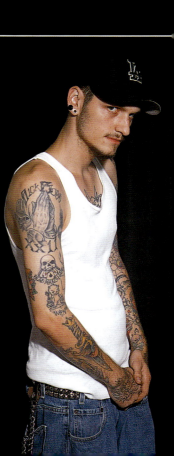

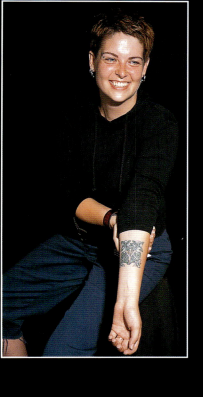
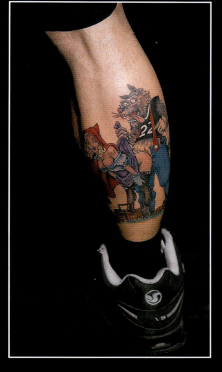
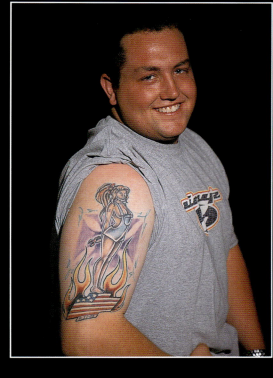

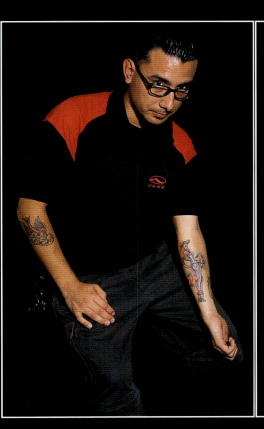
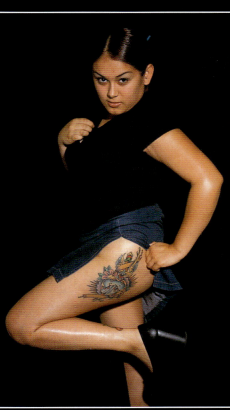
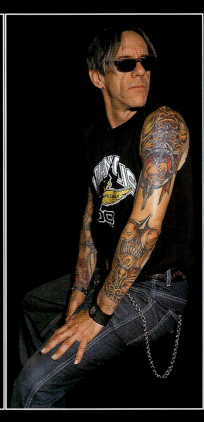

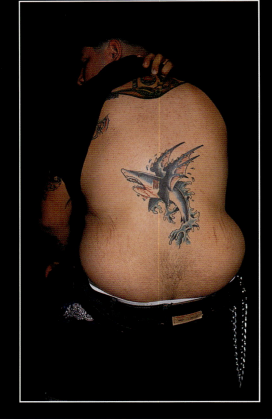

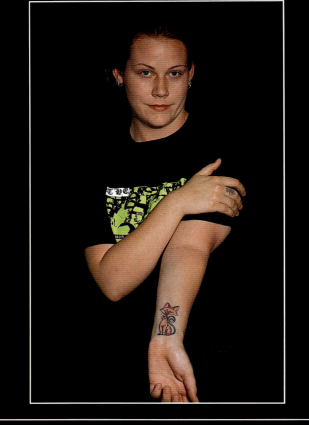

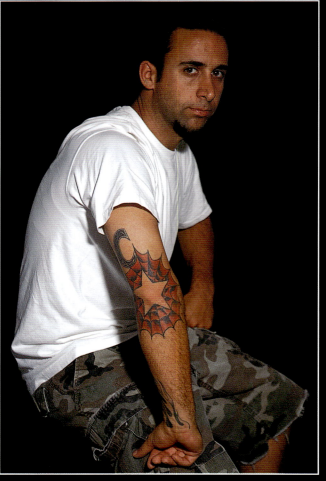

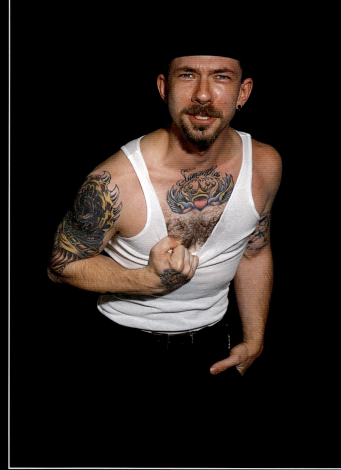

"Jonathan told me all about placement and color schemes. He taught me all about classic Americana tattooing. The way tattoos look, I learned all that from Jonathan Shaw. Whenever Jonathan tattooed, I was there. It was a shop, but it wasn't a walk-in environment. It was appointment only. I hung out for a year and a half, and then, during Christmas of 1991, I returned to L.A. That's when I got involved in the opening of L.A. Tattoo. The first summer of '92, it was me and Baby Ray, Ilia, Jason Brown, Dennis DeGuzman, and Mike Brown. It was a hard-core crew. A good place to sharpen my skills. I knew the Americana tattoos, but my black and gray work and my lettering—I was influenced by Mike Brown. Mike had worked with Ed Hardy. I learned about black and gray from Baby Ray. He was learning too.

"After a while, I had enough of the politics and decided to move. I was working in Los Angeles, and Odie was working at the Venice version of L.A. Tattoo. We decided to open a private studio together. We rented an office building in Burbank—the original Vintage Tattoo. We were there from 1995 to 1997."

A short time later, their names forever enshrined on countless back walls and industrial alleyways, Baba and Odie returned to Highland Park, to the exact same building they used to graffiti when they were kids.

"Our initials are out in front of Vintage on the sidewalk. In the cement from when we were kids. It's like our little home. Now we're the superstars of the neighborhood."

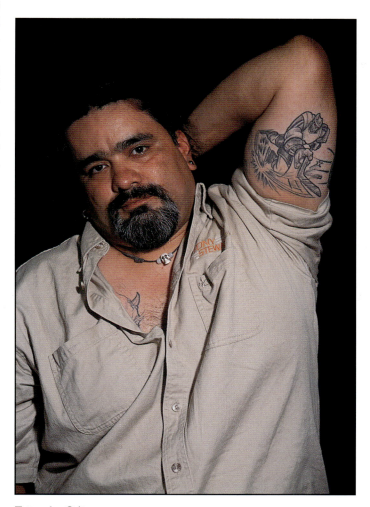

Odie bombs his trademark.

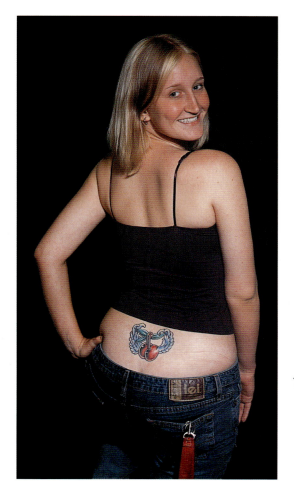

Tattoo by Odie.

Tattoo by Odie.

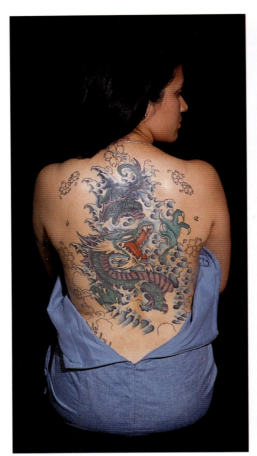
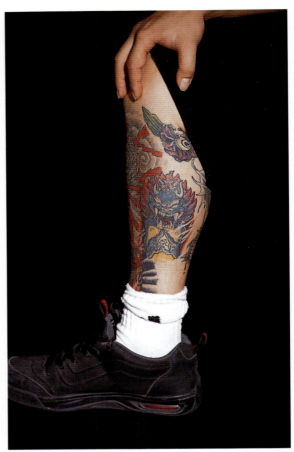

Tattoos by Odie.

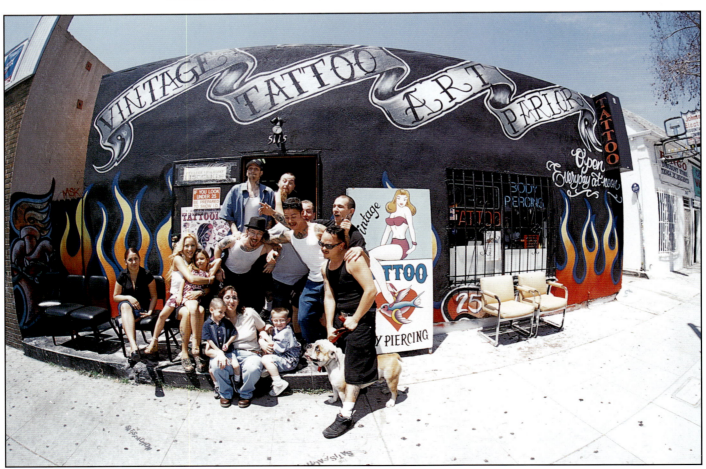

The York Boulevard posse.

DOTTIE M.
TABU TATTOO, MAR VISTA

One of the most beloved and, dare I say, adorable, women in all of tattooing is little Dottie M. Dottie met R.J. Musolf in Minnesota. Dottie and R.J. lived in the same building. Dottie was upstairs with her family, and R.J. was downstairs with his. R.J. was into motorcycles. Dottie was into R.J. They got married and moved to California. Dottie did finances and accounting. When she was 35, Dottie started tattooing.

"I used to do watercolors," she said. "I was always artistically inclined. I was heavily tattooed before I began tattooing. I have always been into tattoos and tattoo shops. I tried to get tattooed when I was a young teenager, but nobody would tattoo me. I talked my dad into taking me to three or four shops in Chicago when I was 15."

R.J. and Dottie left the country for a few months, and, when they got back, Dottie decided to quit what she was doing and apprentice at one of the hottest shops at that time, Sunset Strip Tattoo, with Robert Benedetti. Robert was the first person to tattoo Dottie in 1977. She got a lot of tattoos at Sunset and worked there for three years. Then Dottie and R.J. opened Tabu in 1994. It was

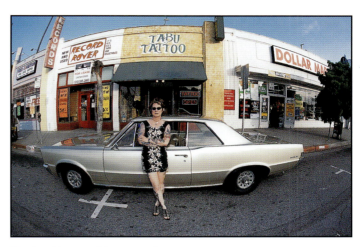

Dottie with one of her great loves.

and is one of the most beautiful tattoo shops in Southern California. R.J. used to be a faux finisher for the casinos in Vegas, which is why Tabu looks so cool. Tabu always has good artists, and one of the best was Dottie M. But Dottie called it quits in 2001.

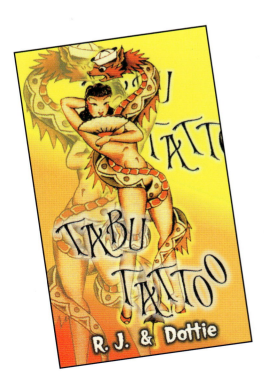

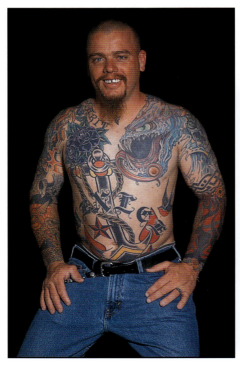

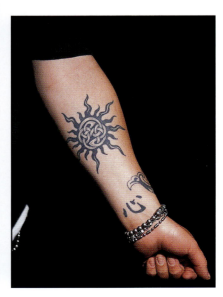

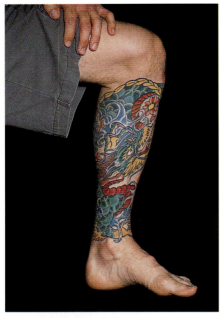

"I tattooed for 11 years, but I had to stop. I have arthritis in my back from a car accident a long time ago. I have arthritis in my neck, and that started bothering me a lot. It was an ongoing problem. Anytime I do anything looking down, I end up with a pinched nerve in my back, and then I can't tattoo for weeks. That's the first issue. Then I developed this tendonitis in my elbow. A lot of artists get it. I did the whole physical-therapist thing. I was trying to work through it for a year. Anybody who does fine detail work can end up with tendonitis. The therapist told me, if I continued tattooing like I was, full-on, balls-out, five or six days a week, I would end up where I couldn't do it at all. I'd do so much damage I'd have to quit anyway. So I thought, *Maybe I'll try to do it part time or a couple days a week.* I did that, but it didn't work for me. It's either work every day or not at all."

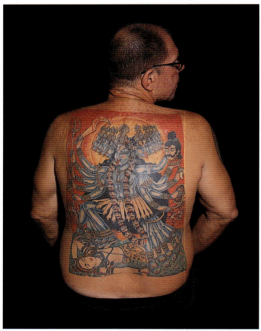

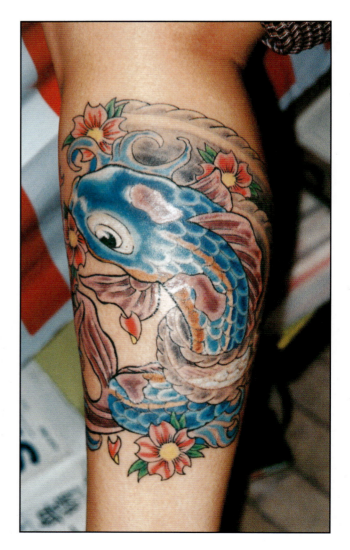

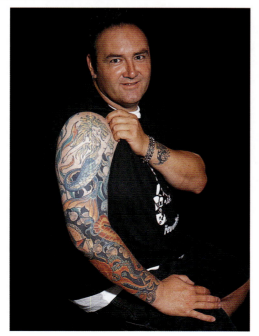

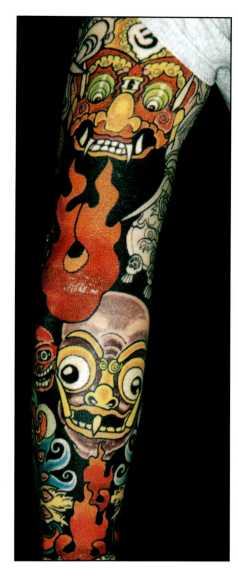
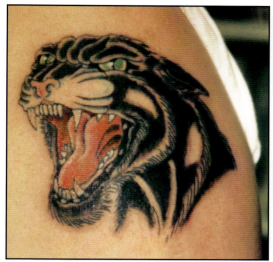
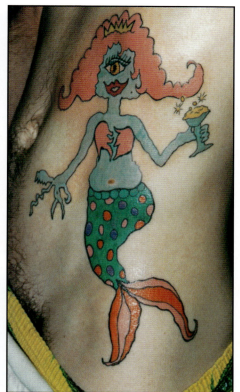
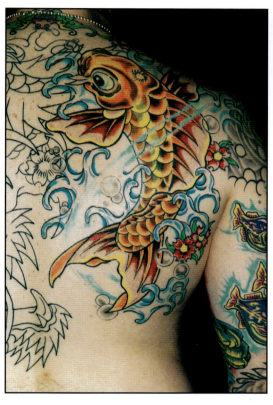
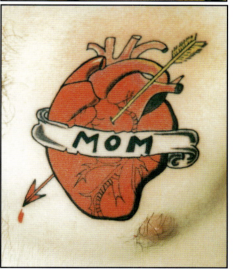

TEARS FOR TATTOOS

"At first, I was really depressed. I cried on the way home from the physical therapist's office. And then I thought, *Quit being such a spoiled brat.* You know, I've had a really good career tattooing. I tattooed for 11 years and was really into getting tattooed. So I finished the ones that were started and started selling machines. I've been really fortunate. I found an alternative way to stay in tattooing and still make a living. I can do something constructive and still be involved with the tattoo community. That's a big part of it for me. It's a whole lifestyle I'll have forever. I even got to go to England and put together machines at Micky Sharpz's. And I'm really into pigment. R.J. and I make all the ink for the shop.

"I've known a lot of people since I started tattooing, and to me I had a super-short career. Eleven years is nothing really, when you think of Jack Rudy, Vyvyn—all these people who have been tattooing most of their lives. Just in my short career, I've seen people start tattooing and quit—start and quit, start and quit, start and quit. People nowadays come in and tattoo two or three years, and say, "That's enough of that," for whatever reason. It's not what they think. But then there's people who have that magic about tattooing. Their heart and soul is in it. Those are the ones who will always be tattooing. They'll always do really well. It's not just a job or making money for them. It's part of your art when you feel that way about it. Those people will always stay in tattooing.

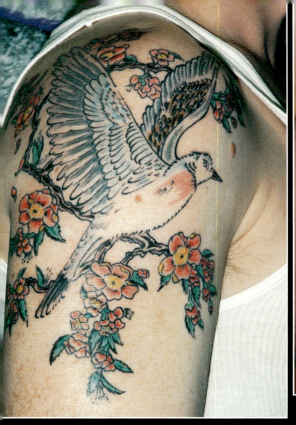

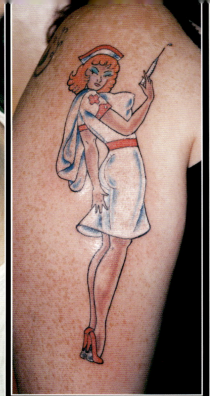

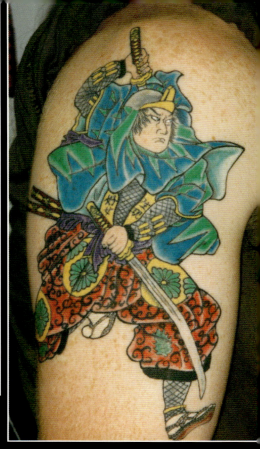

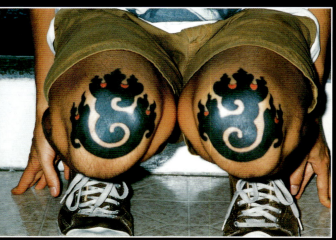

"I believe the future of tattooing is going to come back around. It's changed so much from when I got started. I mean, the reaction to me getting tattooed, it's like night and day compared to 20 years ago. Now it's become the fashion. Like, all of a sudden everyone wants a miniskirt. It's kinda gotten that way with tattoos. Everybody wanted a tattoo as a fashion statement. It's sort of like all fashion: It's short lived. And the people who wore miniskirts because they like to show off their legs, they wear miniskirts their whole life. That's how it will be with tattoos."

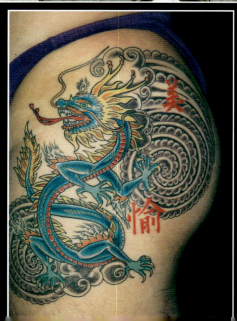

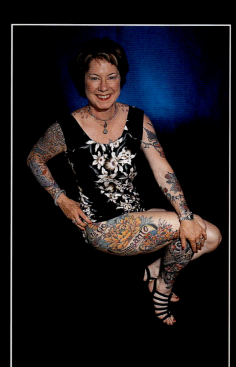

The fabulous Dottie M.

COREY MILLER
SIX FEET UNDER, UPLAND

Just a hop, skip and a jump up the road, Upland's a clean little town about 40 minutes east of Pasadena. Talk about a small town. On a Sunday, there's no traffic, nobody on the sidewalk, and most of the stores are closed. There's a nice bandstand at the end of the main street, but that was empty. Not so at Six Feet Under. The place was humming.

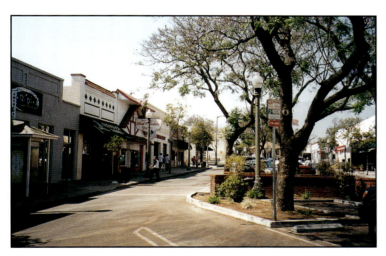

Main Street, Upland.

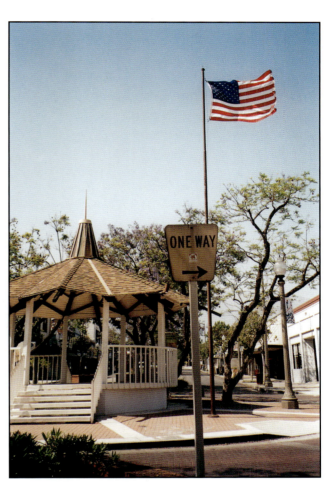

The bandstand at the end of the street.

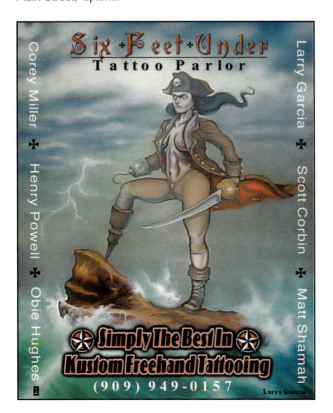

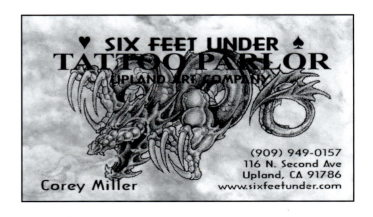

Corey was there with his family, plus three or four other artists working on customers. It's a great-looking shop inside. It had the feel of a fancy, 1890s railroad car.

A well-known musician and tattooer, Corey's from Upland. He inked his first tattoo at 15.

"I got kicked out of class for hand-poking a tattoo on my buddy's arm."

At 16, an ex-con taught Corey to make a machine from a guitar string. It wasn't long before Corey got his hands on a real iron from Spaulding & Rogers.

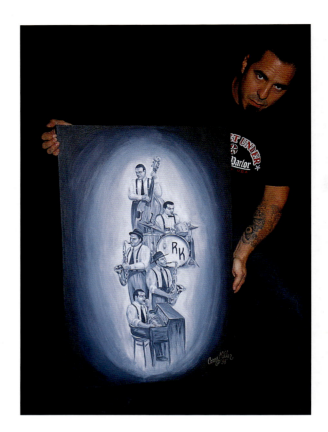

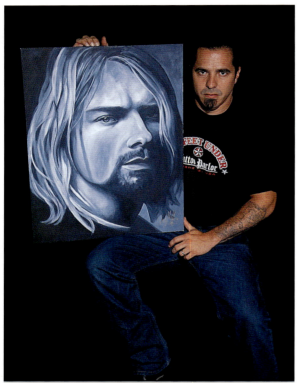

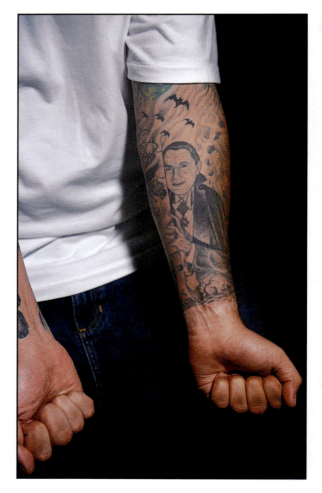

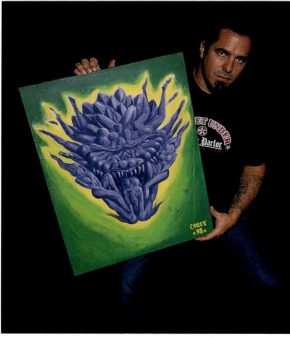

Corey with his paintings.

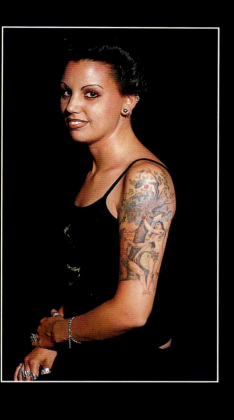
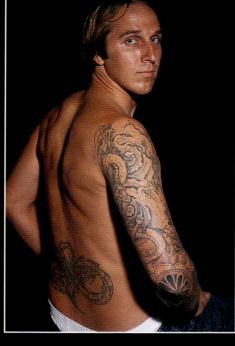
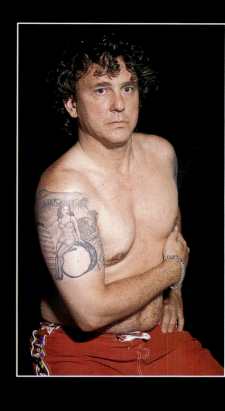
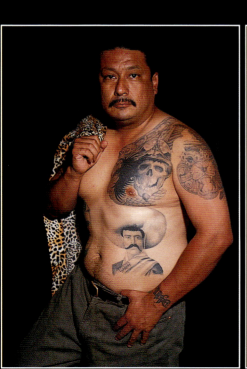
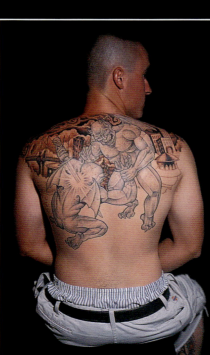
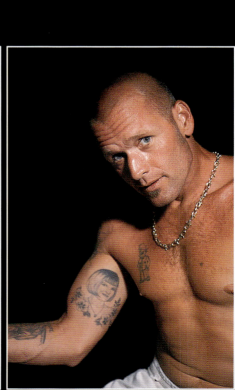

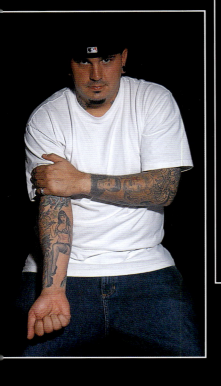

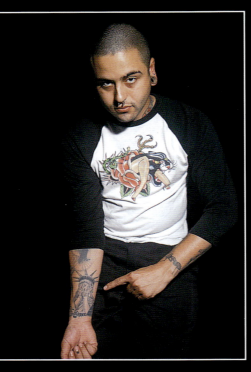

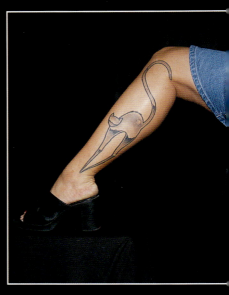

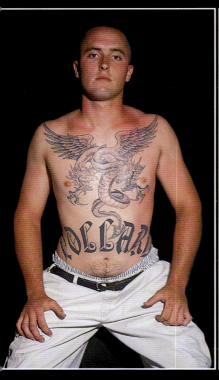

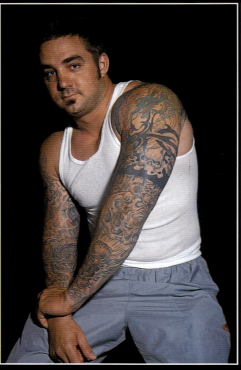

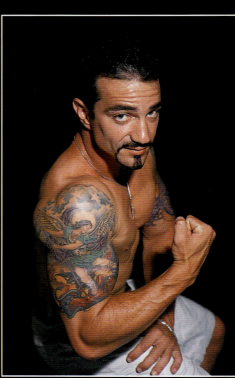

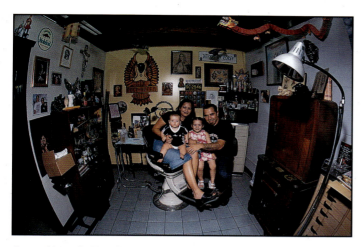

Corey, His wife Kat, Chloe and baby Suzanna.

After high school, Corey's dad taught him finish carpentering. He'd work during the day at construction, come home, party all night and tattoo 'til morning. "I worked out of my house, travel around, hotel rooms, whatever." There was nobody around at that time except Mark Mahoney. They'd go to Hollywood and get tattooed by Bob Roberts. Then Mark hooked Corey up with Fat George at Tattoo Gallery.

"It was a lot scarier back then. Most people didn't want to go to La Puente. I was just a white kid, 20 years old with not too many tattoos on me. It was my very first job. It was busy, like an old Pike-style shop. I was 20 when I started. I'm 35 now. These days you take credit cards. Everything's happy. Everything's nice. It was a much different scene back then."

Corey was there a couple years when Dick Warsocki came in and checked out his work.

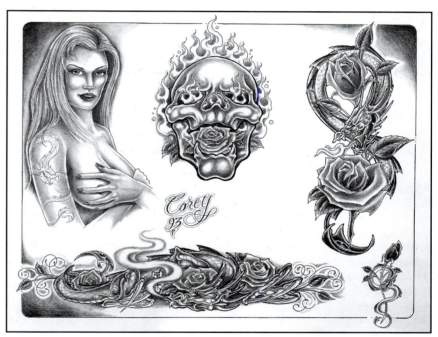

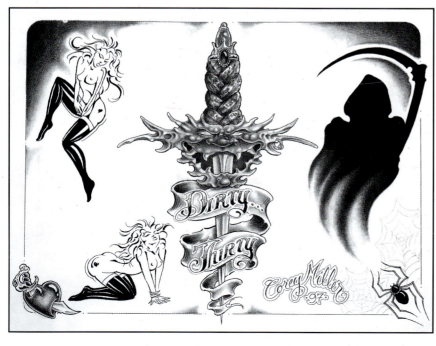

97

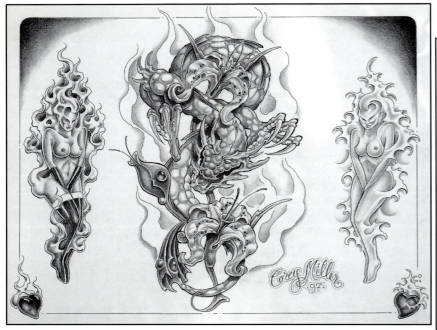

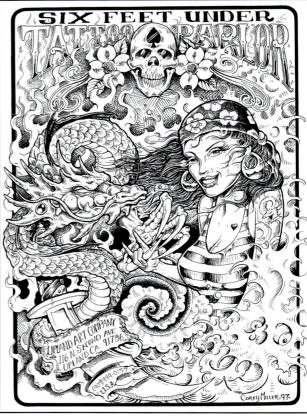

"I was doing this amazing American Indian piece. It was total luck he came in when he did. Dick was really into Indian artwork. He said, 'Wow, where have you been? I've got to take you over to meet Jack Rudy.' That was the transition. Jack told me to quit my job and work for him at Tattooland. That was the best shop I could have gone to. It was my whole upbringing, black and gray, street-style tattooing. I was lucky enough to get involved with people like Mark Mahoney and Jack Rudy right off the bat.

"I worked for Jack a year and a half. Then I got tired of driving around. I knew my town was a hotspot, so in 1991 I opened Optic Overdrive on Central Avenue. Basically, it ended up in gunfire, and we closed down. I was frustrated with what happened with the business and decided to be more underground. So I traveled around—Canada, Hawaii. Then I tattooed in my basement. That got too crowded, so I opened the first Six Feet Under. Then that got really busy. So on April Fools' Day in 1997 I opened up at 116 North Second Avenue."

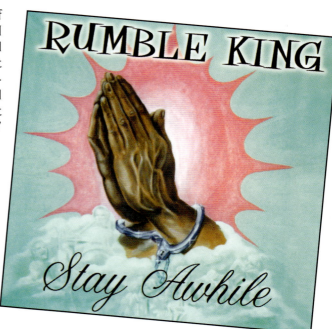

CDs for Corey's band, Rumble King.

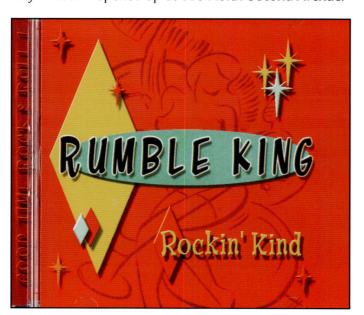

SUZANNE FAUSER

"I can thank a lot of people for influencing me, but the one who really had the biggest effect was Suzanne Fauser. She influenced the whole business. She's the one who said, 'If you act right, you'll last.' Over everybody, she's my favorite. She figured that anyone smart enough to listen to her would learn something. She told me about the great artists I really loved, like Greg Irons. She was so overflowing with knowledge. She went out of the way to introduce me to the right people, which is very rare in this business. She considered me her son. I met her when I was 20 years old and ended up going back to Ann Arbor, Michigan, and working for her for the next 12 years. Last year, when Suzanne passed away, my new baby was born. The highest respect I could give her was naming my daughter after her."

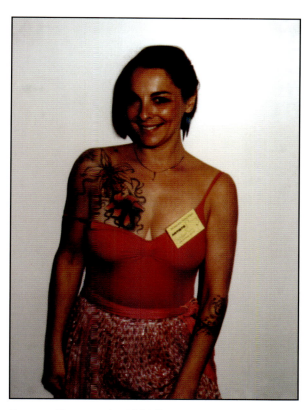

Suzanne Fauser at the 1984 Texas Expo. *Photo courtesy of Tattoo Archive.*

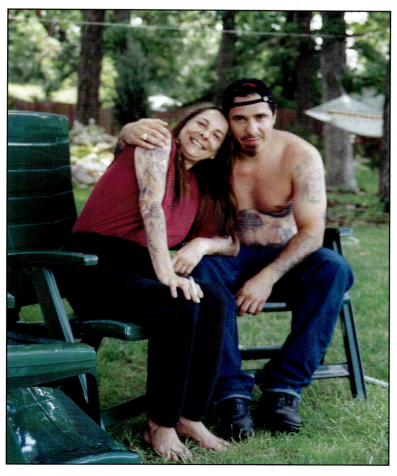

Corey and Suzanne Fauser.

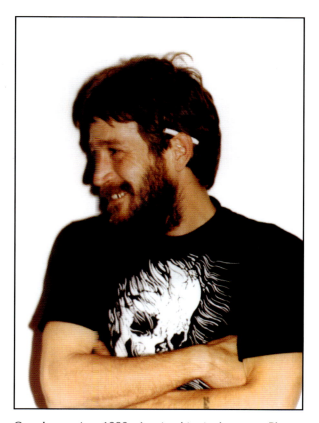

Greg Irons, circa 1980, showing his single tattoo. *Photo courtesy of Tattoo Archive.*

GREG JAMES
SUNSET STRIP TATTOO, HOLLYWOOD

I notice a certain gentleness of spirit whenever I visit Greg James. It's born out of confidence, but not the brash variety so often displayed by certain tattoo tough guys. Greg's strength is in his high level of skill, his almost Zen approach to technique and his humility and grace in accepting the many accolades heaped upon him by a who's who of celebrity clients from Cher to Billy Idol, Mötley Crüe to Courtney Love.

Because it was rush hour, I took the back streets. Far from the glory days when Gilbert Roland and Jeff Chandler drove their top-down convertibles past Schwab's and the Garden of Allah, there's good and bad in Hollyweird. The famous sign is still there and the stars in the sidewalk, but the rest is a mess. Sure, there's no more hookers in front of Hollywood High, and the new Chinese Theatre is pretty spiffy, but for the most part a festering crumminess pervades the place. Everybody talks about bringing back the old Hollywood, but nobody seems to be doing anything about it. Fortunately, tattooing's alive and well on the Sunset Strip. There are four A-listers within five minutes of each other. The most westerly is Tattoomania (currently boasting Freddy Negrete and Jonathan Shaw). The newest of the bunch, Mark Mahoney's Shamrock Social Club, is cattycorner across the street. A couple miles east is Greg at Sunset Strip Tattoo, and a couple doors from that is Purple Panther, owned and operated by the mysterious lady M.

Greg's story unfolds when he was 14. He drew flash for his brother, Tennessee Dave, at Captain Jim's Trade Winds, Seven Seas and 362 on the Pike in Long Beach. Then it was six years at Good Time Charlie's in Whittier.

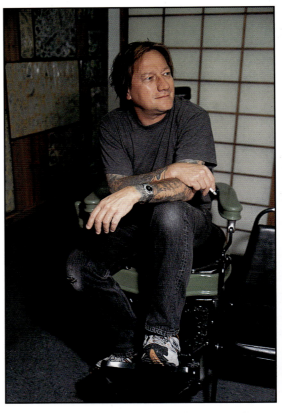

The master, Greg James.

"Basically I was working in East L.A., doing single-needle black and gray. I wasn't very excited about it. I felt I was doing mediocre work, and I wanted to do superlative work. So I made a choice. I would either quit tattooing or try to get in with Cliff Raven at Sunset Strip Tattoo. Cliff hired me. That's the beginning of the story."

BACK IN THE DAY

The original Sunset Strip Tattoo was situated in an area famous for its clubs. The old Ciro's was right across the street. Everybody waiting for a limo saw the tattoo shop. Opened in the 1960s by Lyle Tuttle and sold to Cliff Raven, the new Sunset is about two miles east of the original location. Although many people think it's Greg's shop, Robert Benedetti is the owner. Greg is simply its superstar employee.

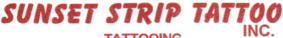

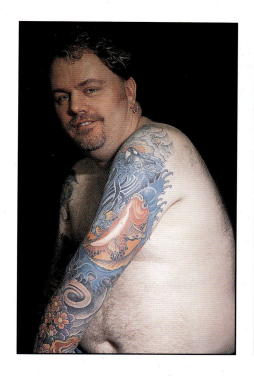
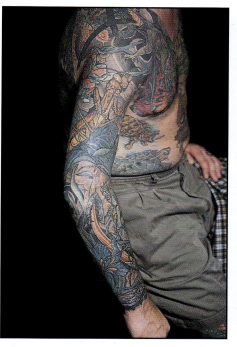
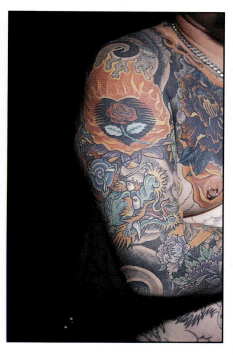
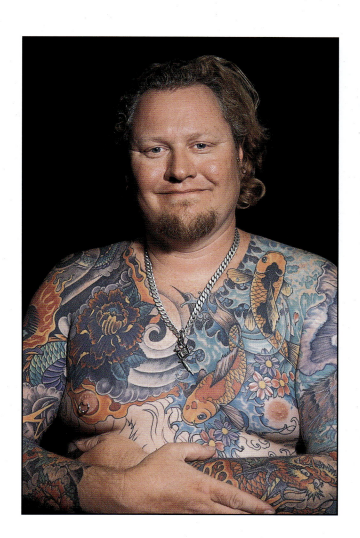
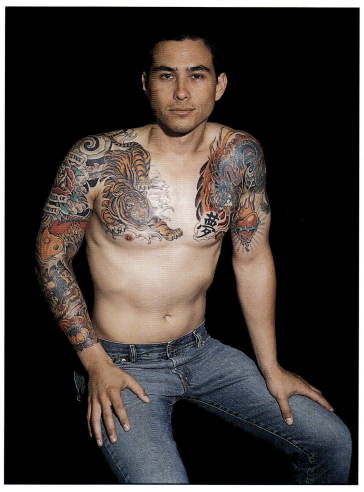

"It's much more freeing that way," explains Greg. "I can just do my work, without the headaches. When I started at Sunset, Robert was the head guy. He took me under his wing. Cliff was in transition. He was living out in 29 Palms and only on premises about two days a week. I got in on the tail end of Cliff being there, when he was moving away, basically. About 11 months after I got hired, Cliff sold the shop to Robert. And Robert continued teaching me.

"Robert showed me about artwork, about placement, about what looks good. The craft, basically. Since then, my style just keeps evolving. I keep polishing it, you might say. I look at other people's work, and I'm influenced by that. All the guys at the shop here, I watch them take a technique, a way of doing things, and make it their own. We all work off each other.

"Working with Robert, I began to understand there is a kind of method, a system. Pigments are mixed a certain way. The power supply and machines are tuned a certain way. They work together in a system. Everybody who works it has further developed that system. It helps with being consistent. When we apprentice people, we teach them that system.

"Traditionally, when you are apprenticed by a Japanese artist, you learn his designs. There is not very much variation. Over here, it's different. I don't believe there are rules. I do it like I see it. For example, I focus more on the subject matter than the background, as opposed to a Japanese tattoo where it's very background-heavy, very dark. I try not to be so dark and so traditional. I don't really follow any rules.

"I've been pretty fortunate. I've been tattooing for some time. Many people have seen my work, and they intellectually decide they want the look I create. Like a lot of artists in this field that are successful, people just tell them to create a tattoo however they want. They might decide on subject matter, whether it's a *koi* fish or a flower or a dragon. They pretty much let you have full control. I think that's the only way you can work. In Japan, for example, when you learn from a master, and you learn his style, you don't deviate from that style. So when you go to that master, you wouldn't ask him to change his style, or do something different. I think people do the same thing here. They see a look that they like, and they don't want to influence that. They want that look. The only way to get it is let the artist do it."

Universally acknowledged as one of America's finest tattoo artists, I asked Greg to give his appraisal of the current tattoo scene—what he thought of the countless new shops and self-proclaimed hotshots entering the scene.

"I really haven't been concerned with what's going on around me," he said. "I just enjoy what I'm doing."

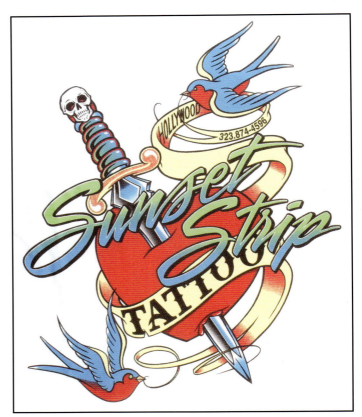

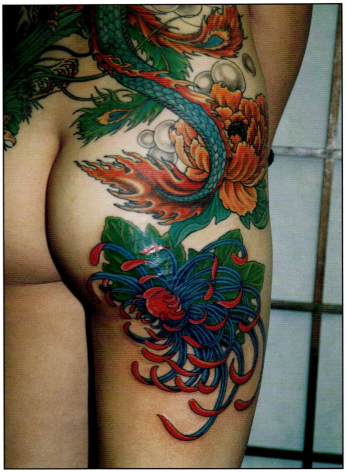

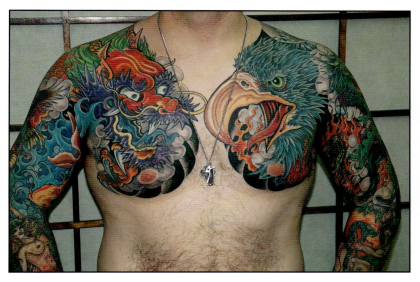

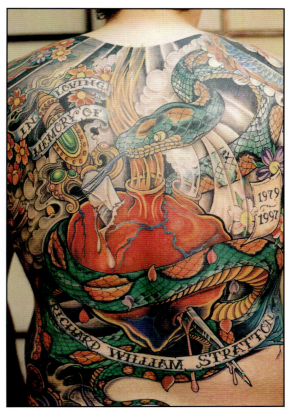

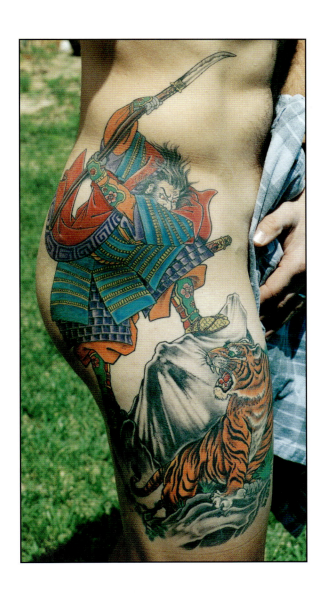

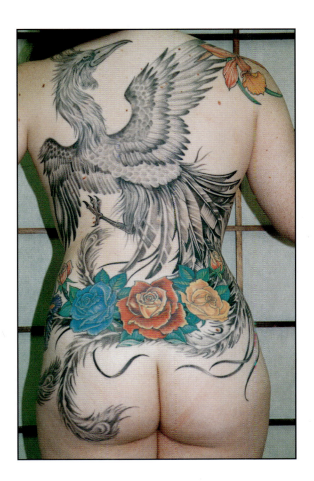

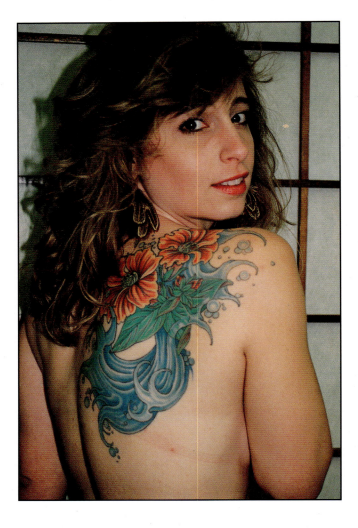

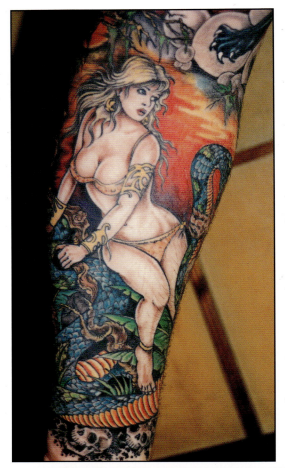

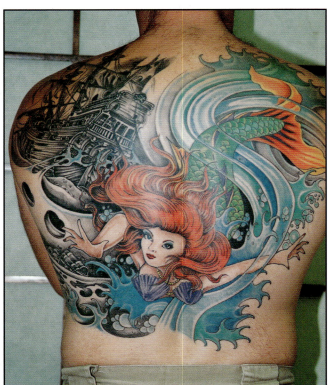

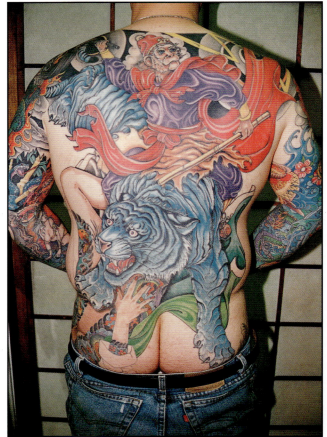

104

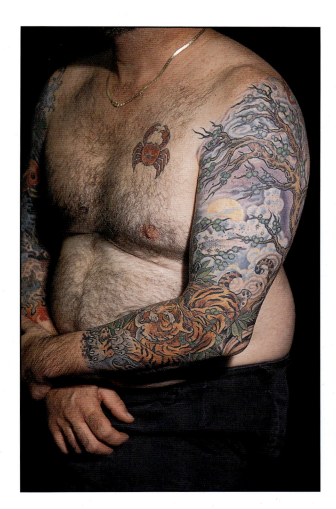

Tattoo by Eric Blair.

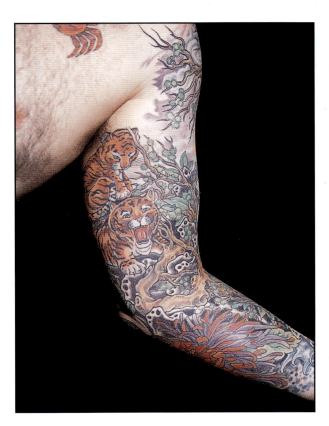

The Sunset crew.

Tattoo by Eric Blair.

PATTY KELLEY
AVALON TATTOO, SAN DIEGO

Back to San Diego again. You know, I've really got to get someone to organize my appointments. Not only am I headed back to San Diego, it's Sunday, and traffic on the 5 has jerked to a halt. It's bumper to bumper at Knott's Berry Farm. Big Fourth of July weekend, and everyone's on the road. It could have been worse. I originally planned to visit Hiro and Maurice Lynch, the old-timers at the oldest shop in San Diego, Masters Tattoo Art Studio on Fifth Avenue, at 11 in the morning, but they cancelled. Funny, I even stopped by and introduced myself to Hiro a week or two before, when I was visiting Dave Gibson. Hiro seemed friendly, but in the interim he and his brother, my links to San Diego's colorful tattoo past, clammed up. They're not the only ones. Joanne Yun, Pinky Yun's daughter who's worked for years on Hollywood Boulevard, and Al at Lefty's in Chula Vista—they all said no.

"Nothing personal," they told me.

For one reason or another, the old guys don't want to rehash the past. It wasn't me. They won't talk to *anybody*! Perhaps it's because they come from a time when artists kept it close to the vest and didn't communicate with people outside their shops.

Damn. But I figured, why blow the weekend? I'll make up for it by visiting two of San Diego's friendliest and most accommodating artists, Patty Kelley and her ex-husband, Fip Buchanan.

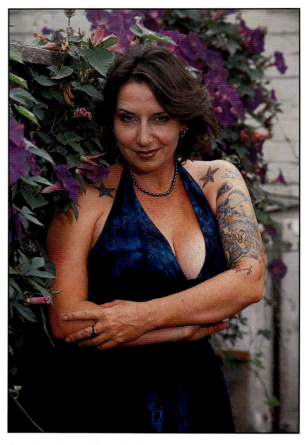

Our dear friend, Patty Kelley.

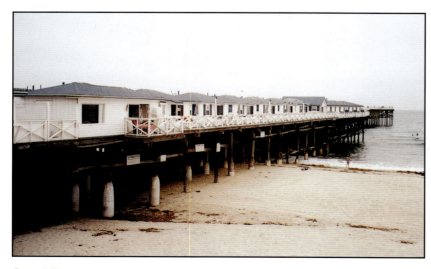

Crystal Pier.

Let's be honest, when you say *ex*-anything in tattooing, expect the fur to fly. But not with Fip and Patty. Every reference to the other was pleasantly couched in the most respectful and loving tone. She thinks he's great. He thinks she's great.

"In fact," says Patty, "I got interested in tattoos and became an artist because of Fip."

Damn, I was hoping for a punch out.

Born in Bridgeport, Connecticut, Patty named her shop for the Avalon Ballroom, a key venue of the '60s rock scene. The Fillmore and the Avalon, that's where Jimi

Hendrix and Janis Joplin started. The famous impresario Bill Graham was a close friend of Patty's father, Alton Kelley. Kelley did posters for Graham and album covers for the Grateful Dead.

I'm living proof that there's *dad genes*," she says.

Patty met Fip when she was 21. They were enrolled at college in Pittsburgh, Pennsylvania, got married and split to the West Coast. Then, after checking out California, settled in San Diego—more precisely, Pacific Beach. Patty's first and only shop was Avalon. She's run it for 13 years.

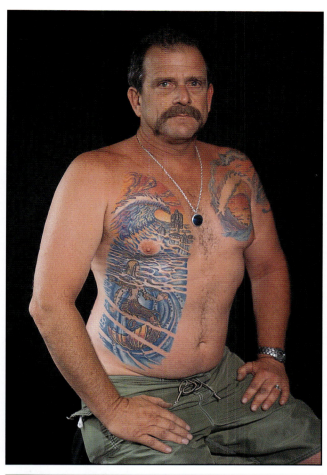

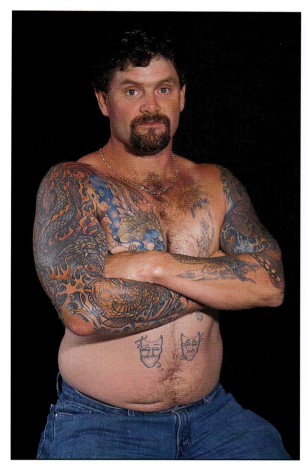

Her friend, David Blackledge.

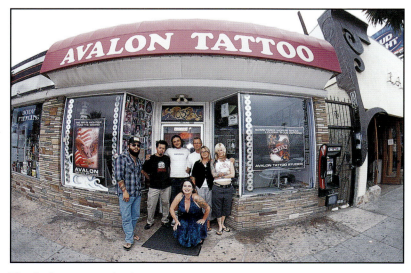

The Avalon guys and gals.

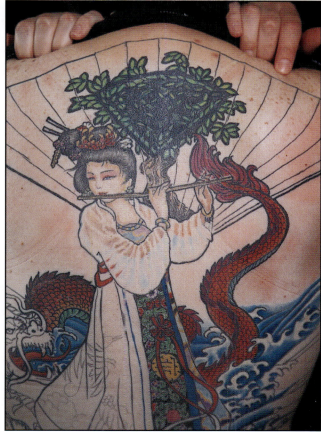

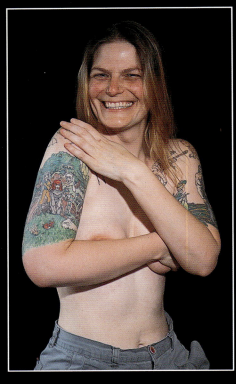
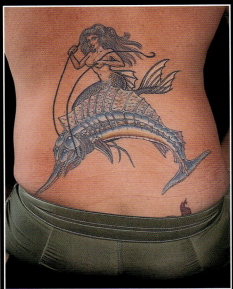
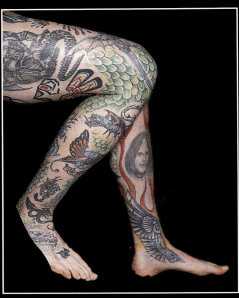
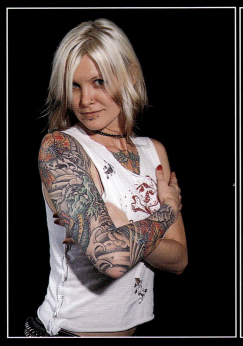
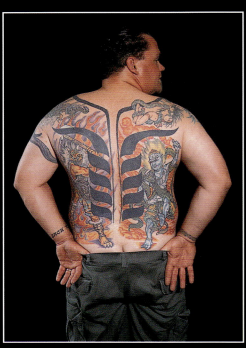
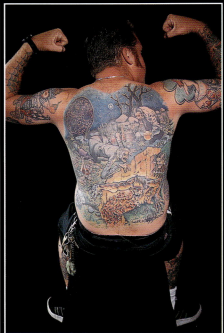

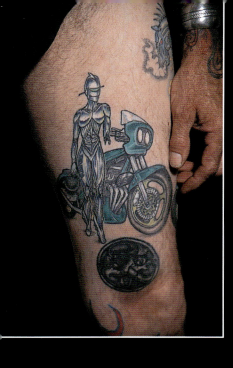
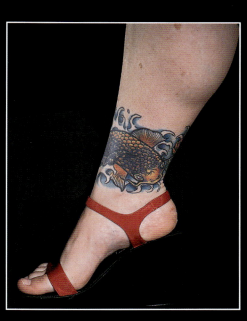
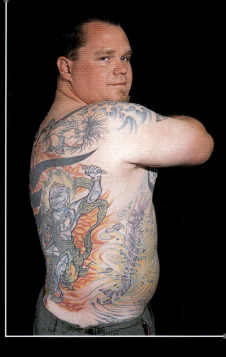
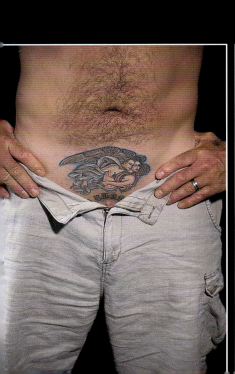
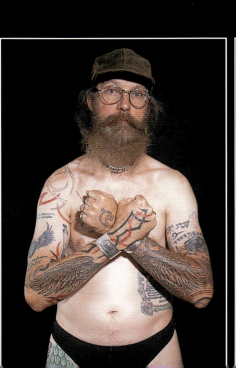
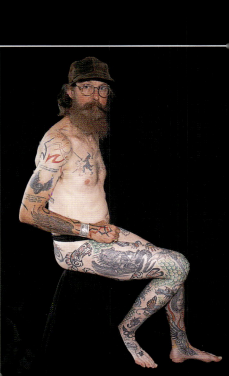

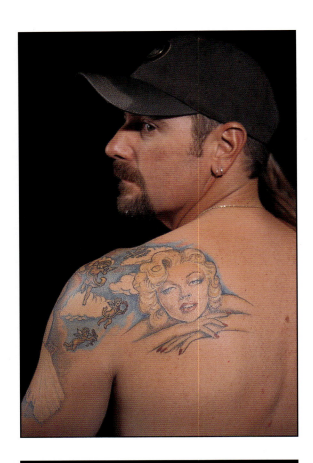

MAJOR INFLUENCES

"When I first got started, I couldn't get any help from the tattoo community. I spoke to Greg Irons before he passed away and all kinds of people. All they said was, 'Yes, dear.' But the more they denied me, the harder I worked. It's the classic story. I'm not the only woman to say this. Back when I started in 1982, the only artists I knew of were Juli Moon, Suzanne Fauser, Vyvyn Lazonga, Patty Pavlik, and Jacci Gresham. I was a big fan. Those five women—it's amazing how many of them were world class. The percentage of women that become top tattooers is well above the percentage for men. It's twice as hard for a woman, so they have to be twice as good. I don't think anything has changed. Remember back when all bank tellers used to be men? The conception was, only men could be entrusted with money. Now bank tellers are women.

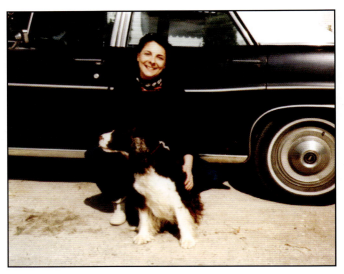

Suzanne Fauser and dog, Jacksonville, Florida, 1983. *Photo courtesy of Tattoo Archive.*

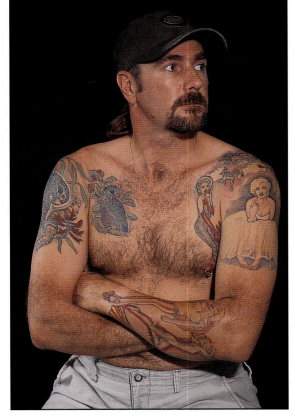

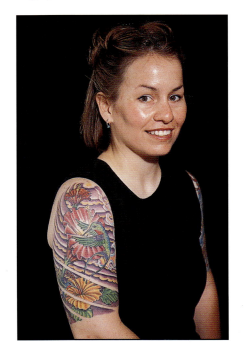

"Recently, I imported some things from Thailand. In order to process through customs, I had to prove who I was, that I owned Avalon. The customs people wouldn't believe I owned a tattoo shop. I had to come up with my business license. If I were a tattooed man, they wouldn't have questioned me. Nowadays, people in the tattoo world treat me with ambivalence, but when I'm with my boyfriend, David, he's the one customers talk to about tattoos. They assume he's the artist. Hell, David's a carpenter. Just because he's a man with tattooed arms, because he's standing next to me, he's the one they talk to.

"The role of women in tattooing has changed considerably in the last decade. For example, I was wearing latex gloves back early on, and I got shunned for it. Wearing gloves! On the plus side, I do think having a woman in a shop is a good idea. It takes the edge off the harshness. With a girl in the shop, you can expect cleaner bathrooms. That attention to detail. And it's not so lascivious. There's a much more comfortable atmosphere. Consequently, more than half our clientele are women.

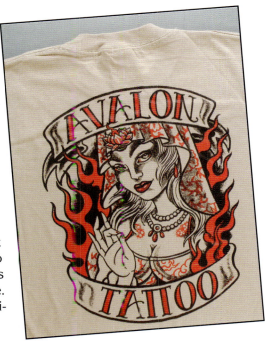

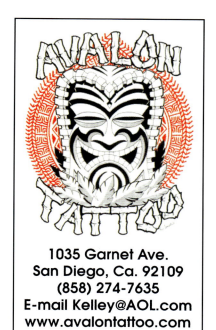

1035 Garnet Ave.
San Diego, Ca. 92109
(858) 274-7635
E-mail Kelley@AOL.com
www.avalontattoo.com

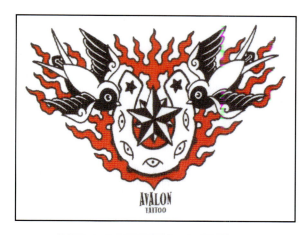

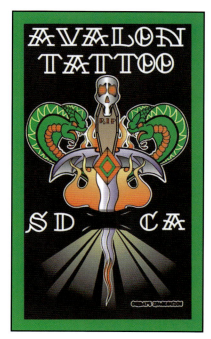

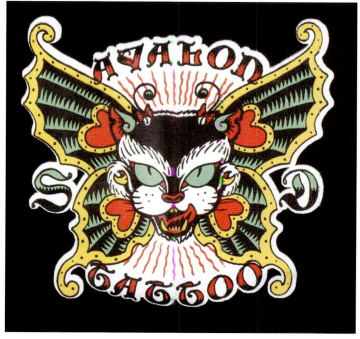

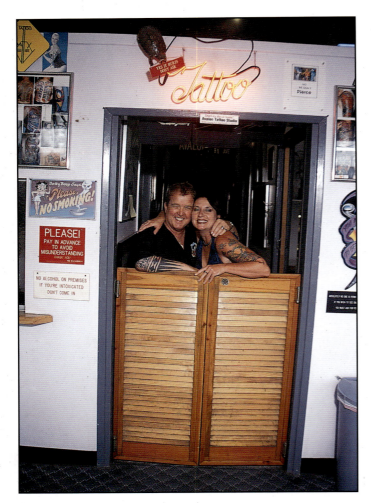

"As for running a business, I can't give you any recipe, but in 13 years, I've had only six employees leave. I must be doing something right. Avalon is the largest shop with the least turnover in San Diego. I'm really proud of that."

By the way, Patty and David took me to the Cass Street Bar & Grill. The gumbo's to die for!

Patty and Baxter.

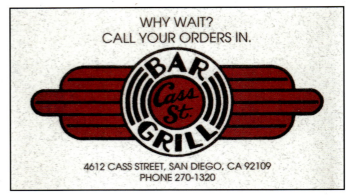

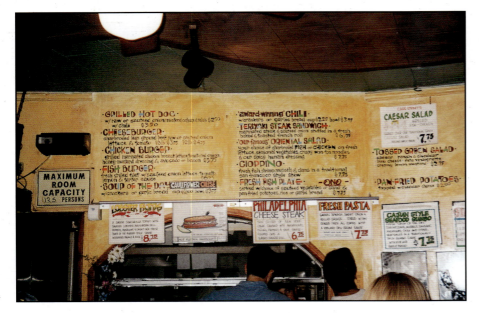

The wall menu from the Cass Street Bar & Grill.

FIP BUCHANAN
AVALON II, SAN DIEGO

It's up the street, get on the freeway, drive east on 8, take the 805 south, exit at Adams—zim, zam, zoom. Just a few minutes away from Avalon I is Avalon II. But the vibe is entirely different. Patty's shop is like a shoe store on sale day, Fip's is more serene, like an art gallery. Open the wrought-iron gate and climb the stairs, Avalon II is white walls, wooden floors, and spotless countertops.

Fip was born in Altoona, Pennsylvania. He caught the tattoo bug at 21. Getting tattooed wasn't very popular back then. It was 1978, and Fip didn't know any shops. He finally found Mike Luckett. Mike tattooed Fip and lent him his equipment, but only after announcing, "Here, take it. I'm going to hell for tattooing people."

Then it was off to art school in Pittsburgh. That's where Fip met Red Schuster. Red tattooed at county fairs. Before long, Fip joined forces with Red and Duke Miller, doing the county-fair circuit. Then Red recommended Fip to J.C. Fly, a Long Island artist headed for Arizona. Fly hired the pair and left four days later. Patty and Fip were left to run the shop in Medford, New York. They had absolutely no experience.

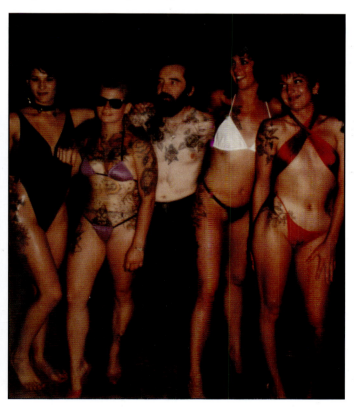

J.C. Fly with friends, 1980s. *Photo courtesy of Tattoo Archive.*

No problem. Patty was very ambitious. She immediately repainted and redecorated the place. But Fly, who had moved to a retirement community in Apache Junction, got fed up and returned about seven months later. Since there wasn't enough work for three people, Patty and Fip moved again. This time to Richmond, Virginia. They ended up running a shop originally started by Danny Fowler. That lasted two years. They finally landed in California, working for Winona Martin. Winona was Jack Rudy's girlfriend. The place was called San Diego Tattooland.

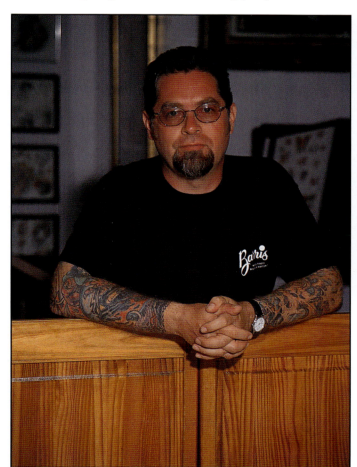

San Diego's own Fip Buchanan.

"When I first arrived," says Fip, "Jack and I were driving by a placed called China Land. It was a Chinese restaurant. Jack says, 'Everything's *Something* Land—*Car Wash* Land, *Auto* Land, *Convertible Sofa* Land. So I wanted Tattooland.' That's how he came up with that name.

"Jack helped me a lot. We'd sit up all night talking about tattoos. He tattooed both me and Patty. I learned a lot just watching what he was doing. It was great, just discussing things. Before that, I never had a lot of direct instruction. When I worked with Red, I'd seen convention photos of work by Jack, Bob Roberts, Ed Hardy and Cliff Raven. They were heads above anyone else. But mainly I learned by getting tattoos."

After a successful stint working side by side with Patty, Fip decided to do a geographic, so they opened Avalon II, about 15 freeway minutes away, some five years ago.

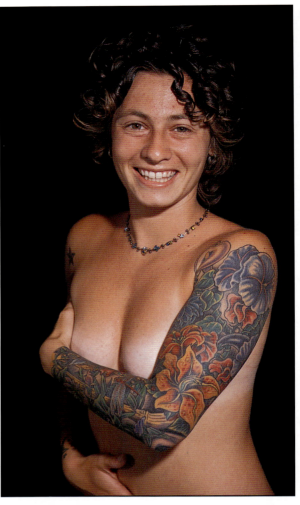

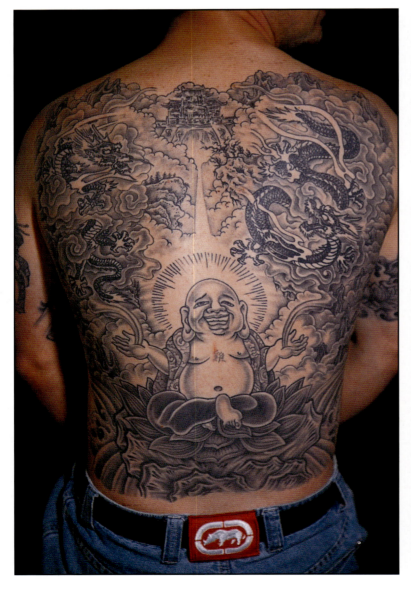

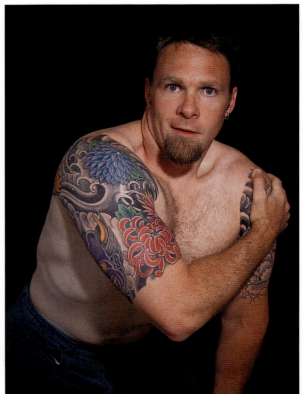

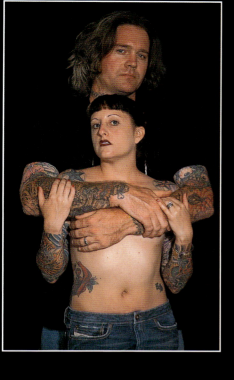
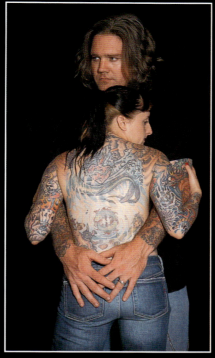
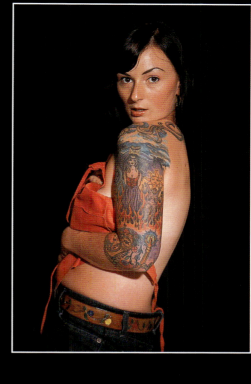
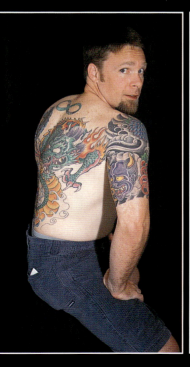
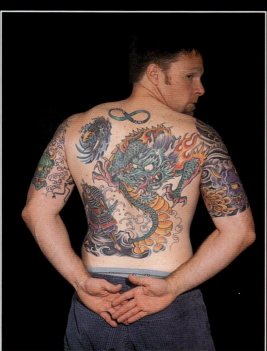
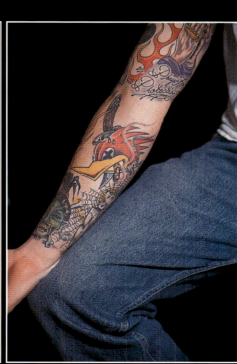

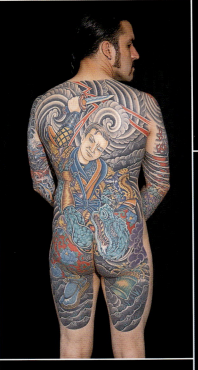
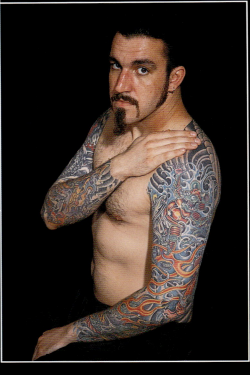
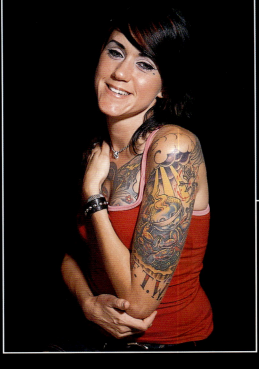
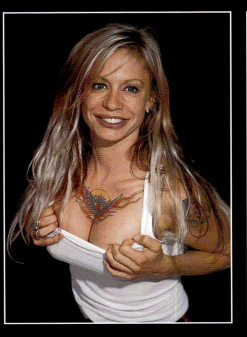
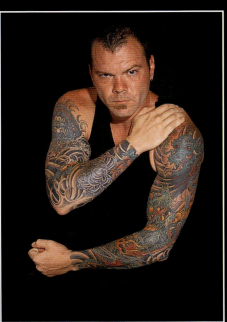
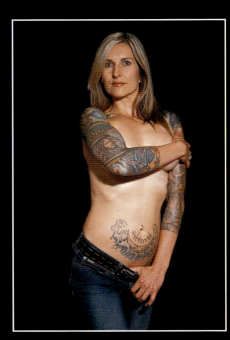

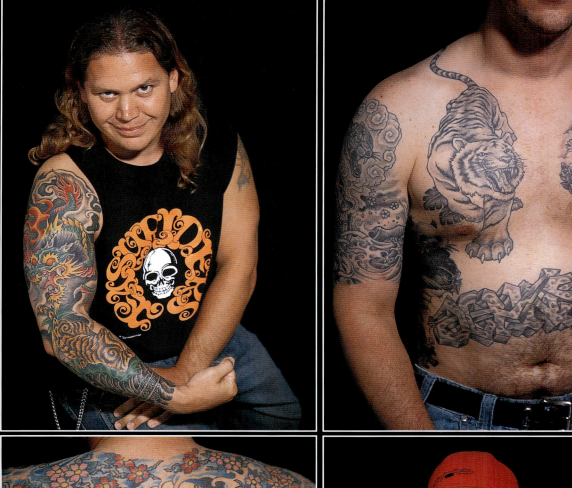
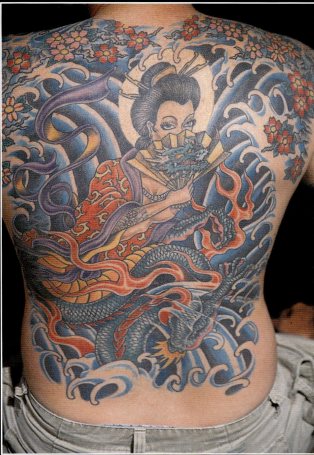
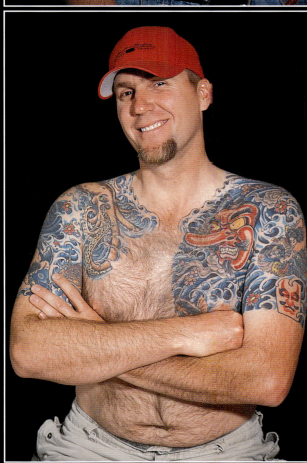

THE CURRENT SCENE

"Nowadays, tattooing is more popular than ever. Everything's so high-tech. People are returning to more primal art, just because it's so nontechnical. And it will continue to become more popular. But, quite honestly, I hope those doing inferior work will have to close their shops, due to lack of business. We're all so convenience-oriented. I have people who come from Arizona and San Francisco, but then there's people who call and ask, 'Where's the nearest shop?' That's all they care about. I wish the clientele would learn to be more selective so only the good tattooist would survive.

"The upside is, because of the popularity, tattoos have become more mainstream. I really like it when I can tattoo a mother and daughter or a father and son, a mother and son, or whatever. I just can't imagine going with my father to get a tattoo. I think it's great. I have a client, I've tattooed both of his sons. I've tattooed his wife through the years. I think it's wonderful that people are so accepting of it now."

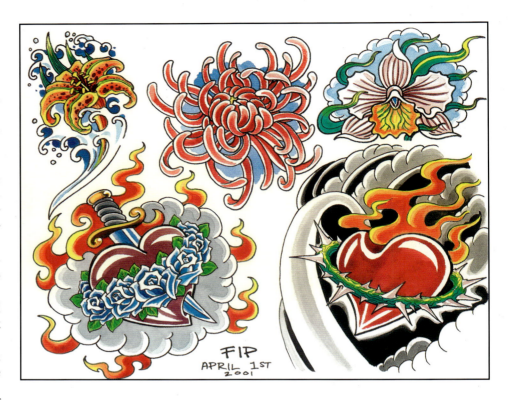

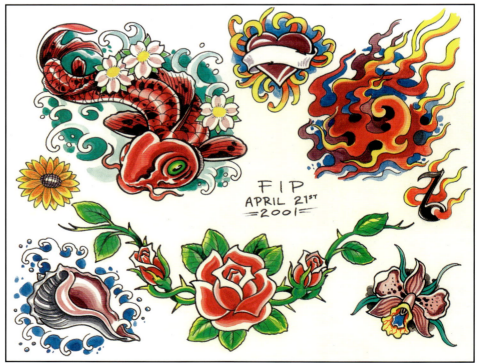

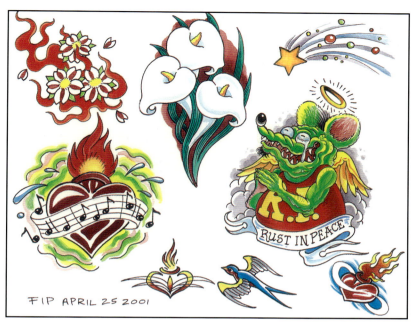

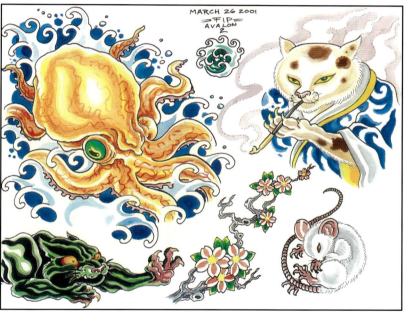

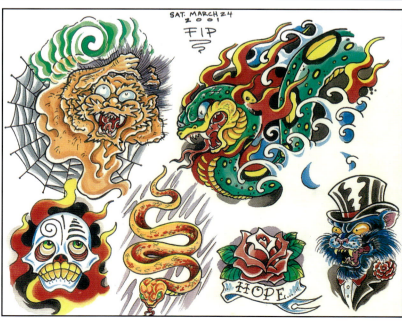

ETHAN MORGAN
SO-CAL TATTOO, SAN PEDRO

Here's a case of nurture vs. nature for you. The immensely talented Ethan Morgan, the prize-winning tattoo artist at SoCal Tattoo in San Pedro, just like Patty Kelley at Avalon, has a famous commercial-artist father.

"My dad is pretty well-known in the animation field. He's worked for everybody—Disney, DreamWorks, Hannah-Barbera, all the major studios. His name is Don Morgan. Every kid wants to be like his dad. I remember him bringing work home every night. I'd grab a piece of paper and a pencil, sit on the floor and draw along."

Another case of *dad genes*, just like Patty Kelley? There's one significant difference: Ethan was adopted.

"My dad's very proud of me. Both he and my mother have given me a lot of support. He's happy that I'm making a living with art, even though, he said, tattooing's permanent, and his pencil has an eraser on it. My parents always encouraged me. They were the first ones to say, 'You don't have to have a job you hate. You can have a job that you love.'"

Dottie and R.J. from Tabu Tattoo recommended Ethan. "He's perfect for your book," they said. That was good enough for me. But I'd never met Ethan and wasn't familiar with his work. I hadn't a clue who he was, but what the heck. Time to take the 110 south.

I arrived at the plain-Jane San Pedro strip mall in less than an hour. From the outside, SoCal is easy to miss. It's clean and clutter-free, like they moved in Tuesday. Decorated primarily with trophies for 1st Place Black & Gray and Best Tattoo in Show, the shop is mainly white walls and fluorescent lights. Funky it's not. When I entered, Ethan was finishing an armpiece.

"I'll have it done in time for a photo," he assured me. On the counter was his book of samples. I took a peek. Righteous stuff. I've seen a million black and gray, jailhouse tattoos. Most of it second rate. There's only a few great black and gray masters—Jack Rudy, Paul Booth, Freddy Negrete. Very few excel. From what I saw, Ethan Morgan was an artist to be reckoned with.

"I always liked to draw. That's what I did in my spare time. I was primarily a musician. A guitar player, singer. That is what I really wanted to do—the Hollywood dream. That didn't pan out, but I didn't actively become a tattoo artist. In fact, I wasn't sure I'd be particularly good. Eleven years later, here I am."

The story goes that Ethan's wife, Terri, was getting tattooed, and the artist offered *her* an apprenticeship. Terri said no.

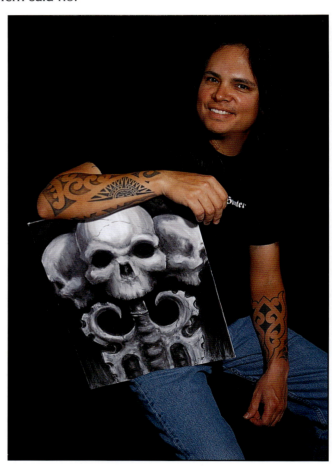

Ethan Morgan from San Pedro.

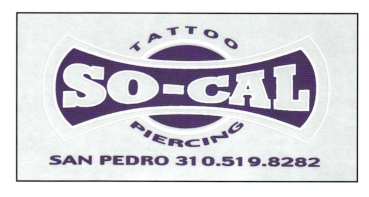

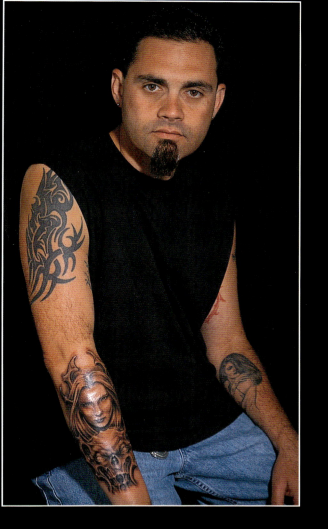

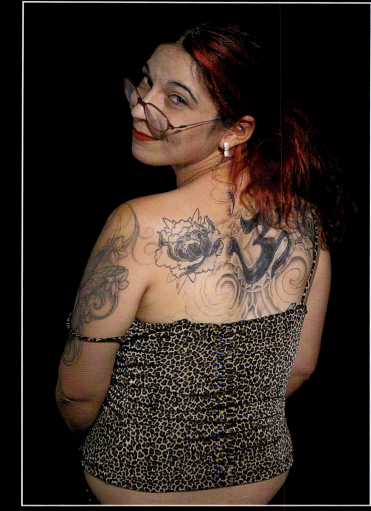

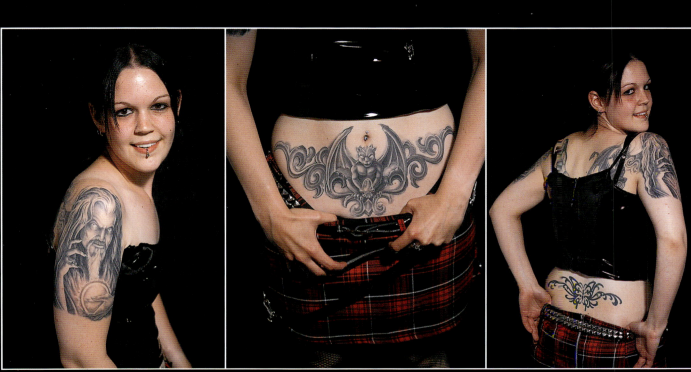

121

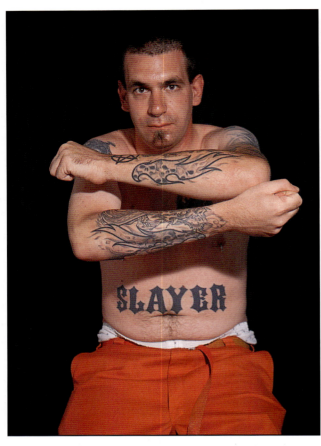
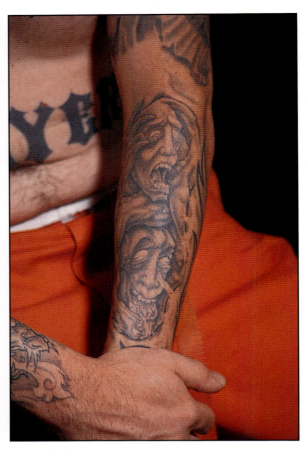
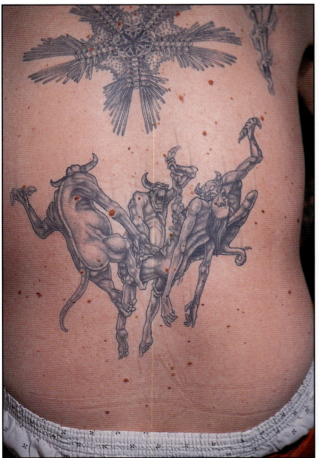
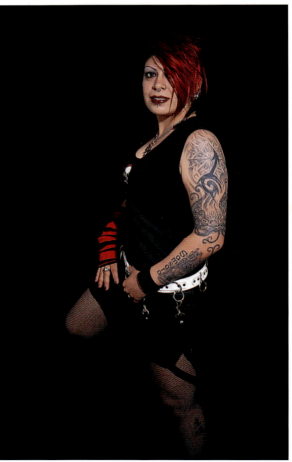

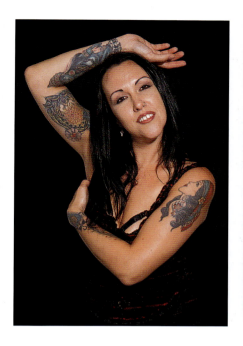
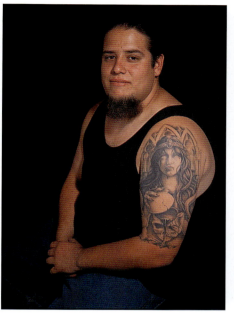
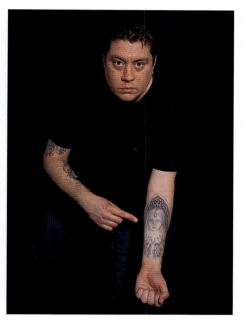

"So I got offered the job," said Ethan. "His name was Steve Saller. 'Pop' Saller. He said I'd be an idiot if I didn't do it. He used to work under Captain Jim on the Pike. His health was failing, and he wanted to pass something on. The shop was called American Tattoo. It was a good, old-fashioned, toilet-scrubbing, cleaning-the-alley apprenticeship. I sterilized equipment, made needles and drew for everyone in the shop. A lot of the guys who worked there didn't draw very well. They needed someone to come up with designs. It was very old-school. One day I came in, and they said, 'Today you put on your first tattoo.' It was like those old-timey apprenticeships you read about.

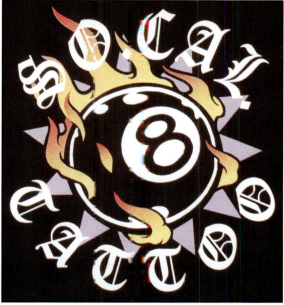

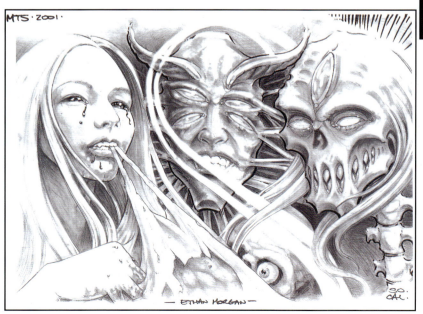

"But it wasn't just about mopping floors. Pop taught me a lot about life, how to deal with people. How to deal with yourself, as well as the tattooing. He helped center me and make me a man. At that time, I was married with kids, but I was still trying to do the whole Hollywood scene. He grounded me and helped me realize I needed to grow up and take care of business. The apprenticeship program is the only way to go.

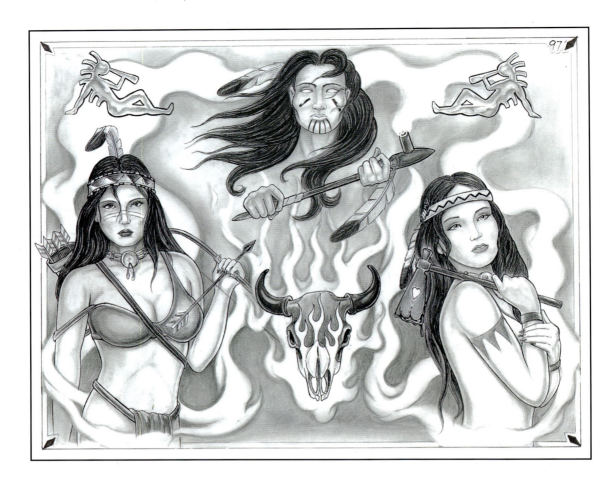

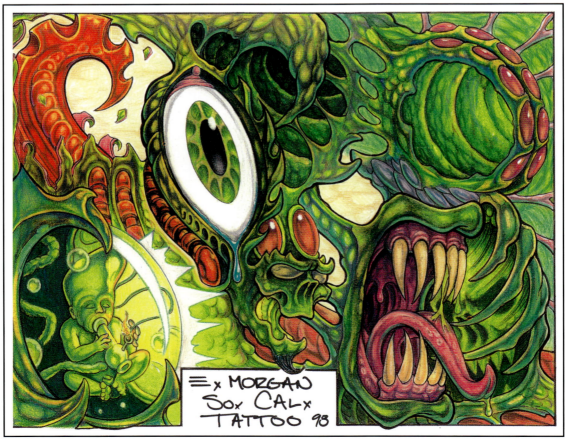

Ξ× MORGAN
Sο× CAL×
TATTOO 93

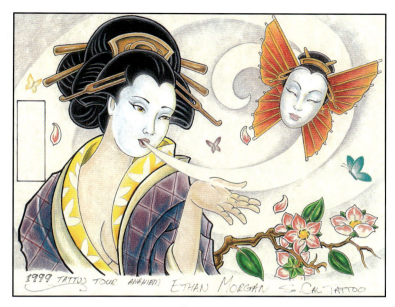

"It wasn't easy. Pops was also one of those guys that, if I didn't do it, if I wasn't getting any better, he wouldn't teach me anymore. I watched two or three other guys get booted out because they didn't evolve, they didn't get better—or they didn't have the artistic talent to get better. He was really hard on me. At the end of the day sometimes, he would bust my chops. There were days I wanted to smash the place. But when I got home, I realized this guy is teaching me to be a tattoo artist. He really taught me a lot."

LEAVING THE NEST

After a year and a half at American, Ethan decided to move on. He looked everywhere for a location.

"You have to go all the way up to Venice to find a beach city that allows a tattoo shop. We were ready to pull up stakes and work for a friend of mine in Chico, but my wife reminded me that she was born and raised in San Pedro. So we toughed it out and stayed.

"I've had over 20 jobs, and tattooing is one of the strangest businesses I've ever been involved in. It's strange, because it affects people. You're doing something that is indelibly changing someone for the rest of their lives. There were times it was like a assembly line. It got to be a blur. I stepped back and realized, people don't understand how deep it is. You're tattooing people because they're making a statement. Or seeking closure. Or they're getting tattooed to cement who they are, where they came from, what they're all about. As a tattoo artist, you're there to help them out. To make their feelings, their thoughts, become a reality. I admit that sometimes it's just a job—doing hearts and banners, but sometimes the customers are on a different plane. They appreciate the time, the insight and the vision that goes into the artwork. Those are the people that I love tattooing. Everyone that you're photographing here today is like that."

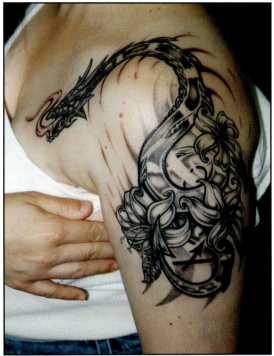

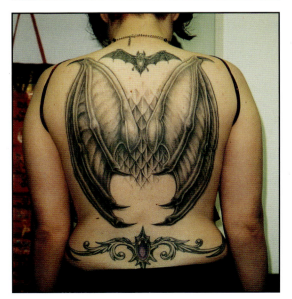

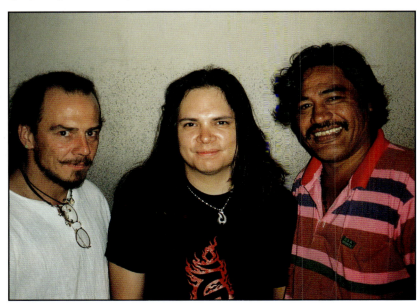

(l. to r.) Mo'o, Ethan, and Petelo Sulu'ape in Madrid

STEVE SMITH
THE ACE TATTOO, OCEAN BEACH

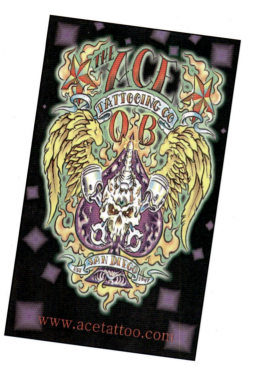

www.acetattoo.com

It's very important to keep up one's strength. This is why, on yet another visit to San Diego, I exited at Capistrano. Home of yet another Father Serra mission, San Juan Capistrano is the humble host to thousands of tourists bent on capturing the famous flocks of swallows that return each year with their disposable cameras. Actually, it's the *tourists* who have the cameras, *not* the swallows. In any case, we're not here to see no freakin' swallows. We're here for lunch. And not some quickie burger joint or tony tourist trap with damask tablecloths and five kinds of margaritas. No, it's time for El Maguey, home of some truly radical *carnitas*. That's slow-cooked pork, baby. The shredded kind that melts in your mouth. Big, juicy hunks of pork, gently tugged from the roast by the delicate hands of brown-eyed, Castilian virgins—the skin still on, all crisp and brown. The *pork,* not the virgins. With plenty of *refritos*. The home-style kind, all caramelized and sweet. And mounds of *picante* Spanish rice—fresh-chopped onion and fragrant cilantro on the side. Plus, a steamy stack of fresh flour tortillas. Whoa, *madre!*

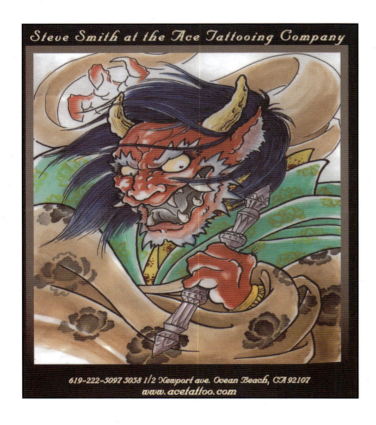

Steve Smith at the Ace Tattooing Company

619-222-5097 5058 1/2 Newport ave. Ocean Beach, CA 92107
www.acetattoo.com

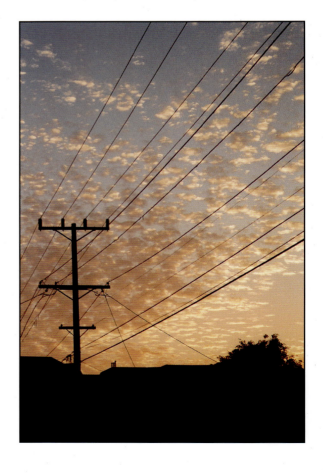

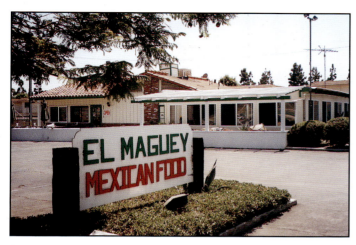

Smell the cilantro?

My *tomar un luncheon* completed, it was on to Ocean Beach. And I wouldn't be in Ocean Beach if it weren't for Fip Buchanan. When the Lynch brothers decided not to be interviewed, Fip called Steve Smith, tattoo artist at The Ace. This was so typical of my road trip: one pal referring another. The natural process of meeting new friends in the world of tattooing. So, instead of being hung up, I'm talking to a guy who's more than happy to share his memories of the historic San Diego tattoo scene.

Born in Tomahawk, Wisconsin, Steve could draw anything he saw. He was 16 when a cousin returned from the Navy with a Buddha tattooed on his belly (they shared bellybuttons).

"It was the coolest thing I ever saw," says Steve.

From a military family, Smith enlisted at 17, arrived in San Diego and, two weeks later, got his first tattoo from Tahiti Felix Lynch at Masters. Talk about six degrees of separation! Felix Lynch is Hiro and Maurice's father. Remember, they were the brothers who wouldn't be interviewed?

Anyway, when Steve Smith was a teenager, the center of activity was lower Broadway, the downtown area from Horton Plaza, Fourth or Fifth Avenue to the pier. At various times in the '40s, there were ten, maybe a dozen shops up and down the street. During the '60s, five or six. There was a renaissance toward the end of the '70s—ten maybe 12 shops in the first two blocks. That's when Steve started. He's been at The Ace Tattooing Co., the shop with the neon sign designed by Zeke Owen in 1969, ever since.

"My first boss was Crazy Bob Silas," he told me. "Crazy Bob was around for about six months. Then Inker Ron Howell. He was trained by Don Nolan and Bob Shaw. I worked for Ron the longest. Gary Hoag bought the shop in '91. The shop's been in Ocean City since '87. The reconstruction and redevelopment started about 1985. By approximately '86 or '87, almost all of the shops were gone from downtown. They were trying to revitalize the business district and expand the tax base. Where our shop used to be is a building that takes up an entire city block."

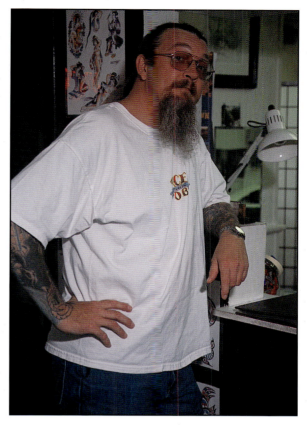

Tattooist, historian and all-around good guy, Steve Smith.

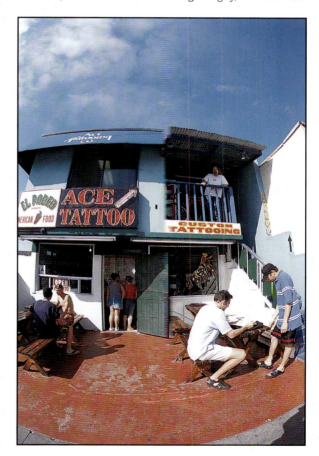

The shop overlooking the beach.

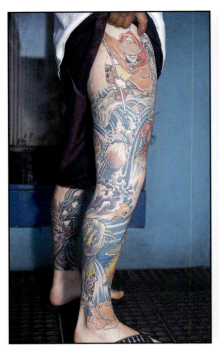
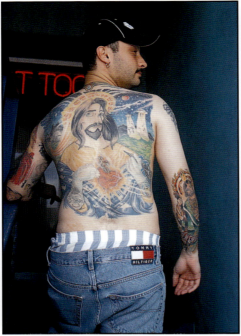
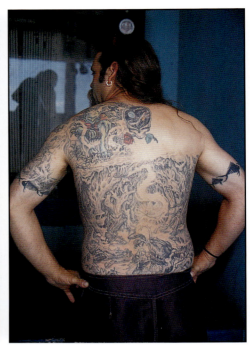

BEFORE THEY TORE IT DOWN

What about the old-time tattoo artists?

"Doc Webb is one of the most famous. He tattooed around the world. I saw a photo of Doc Webb standing next to Tahiti Felix in front of a sideshow poster in Hawaiian-style clothing. That had to be from the late-'20s or early-'30s. I know Doc opened his shop, Old Doc Webb's, in the mid-'50s in downtown. There was a shop called Steamer's Lane, I remember that one. It was on Broadway, right where the new courthouse is now. The guy who owned it got run out of town by the bad element sometime in the mid-'60s. There was a light criminal element involved with some of the tattoo shops in the late-'60s and early-'70s. Not anything heavy. Massage parlors and the like. Masters opened in the late-'40s. That was Tahiti Felix's place. The original Masters was across from the Greyhound bus station down on First.

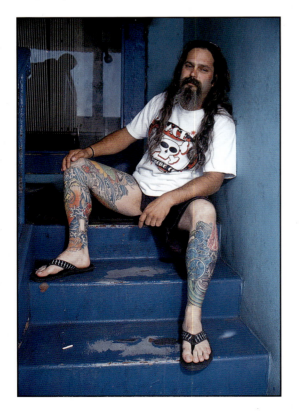

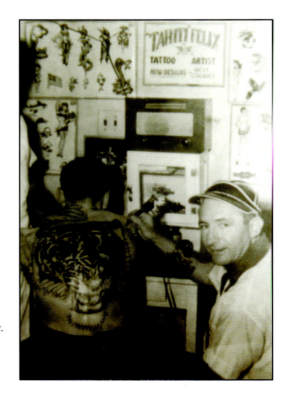

Tahiti Felix Lynch with backpiece, 1950s. *Photo courtesy of Tattoo Archive.*

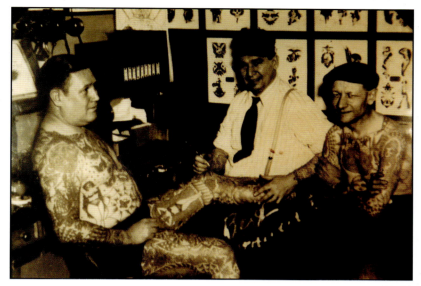

Bert Grimm tattooing, Saint Louis, Missouri, 1940s.
Photo courtesy of Tattoo Archive.

"Then, of course, Painless Nell, her sister, and Painless Nell's husband. They ran three or four shops in the downtown area. Their shop at 348 West Broadway became The Ace. Bert Grimm had a shop, a place called the Illustrated Man. There was a guy named Trader Jim Kunkel in the '60s. Ed Hardy worked for Mike Malone at The Ace. I don't know who actually owned the shop at the time. I don't know if it was Zeke Owen or not, but Ed worked for Mike Malone for a while and opened up his first street shop here in San Diego called the Ichiban."

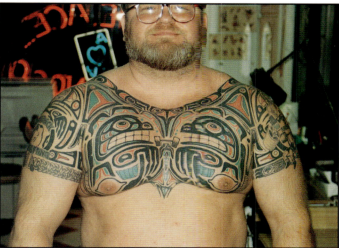

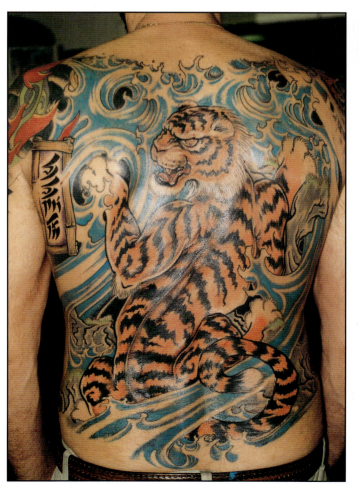

When I think of San Diego, I think of military tattoos.

"That was what San Diego was all about for about 50 or 60 years, until the reconstruction forced everyone out of business. We looked forward to the first and 15th of each month. Sailors were out there looking for a good time on a limited budget. They went to the downtown area. There were tattoo shops and massage parlors, arcades and locker clubs. At one time, you couldn't leave the military base unless you were in uniform, so you kept a locker in town with civilian clothes. When you come off base, you'd go to the club, change into your civvies and go around town. You didn't want to look like the young military guy waiting to be ripped off. It was quite the fun time in the '70s. A lot was going on. When we moved out of downtown in 1987, there were only two shops open in San Diego: The Ace and Masters. There were no other shops. Today, there are more shops in San Diego than there's been in the history of the city. I can't believe the proliferation. Somewhere between 40 and 45 in and around San Diego. There's definitely a renaissance."

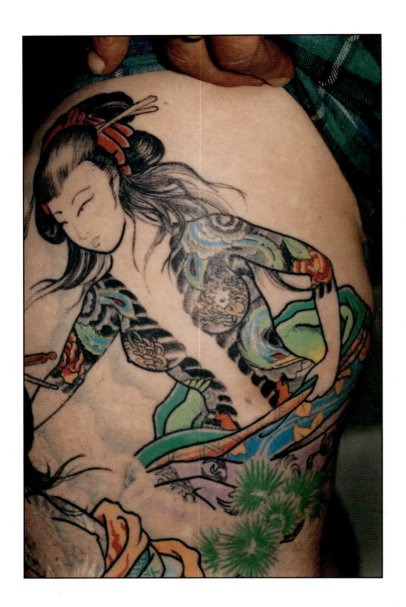
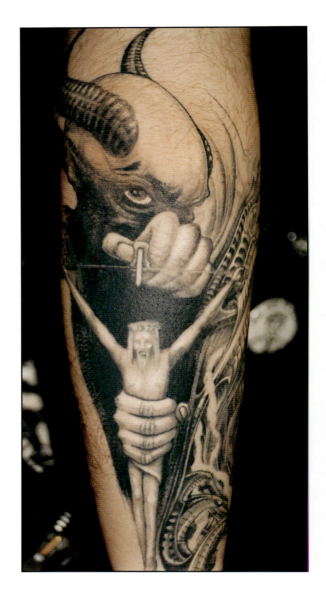

I liked talking with Steve. The shop was jammed with people. It was the kind of old-days energy I remember as a kid. When tattoo shops were dens of iniquity in downtown San Diego.

EMELIO CUSIDOR &
KERRI HODSDON
SACRED ART TATTOO, GARDENA

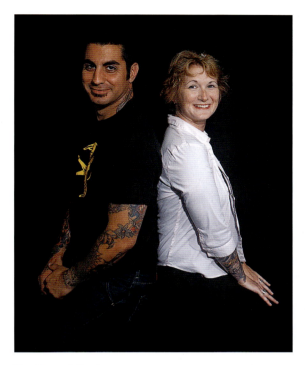

Emelio Cusidor was born in New York, raised in Los Angeles. His Cuban parents moved to the South Bay when Emelio was one year old. Always the artist, Emelio latched onto the typical "three-year apprenticeship where you suffer and clean a lot" at Robert Silva's Norwalk Tattoo. His first job tattooing was at Dave Orlowski's Long Beach Tattoo. The shop did mostly black and gray.

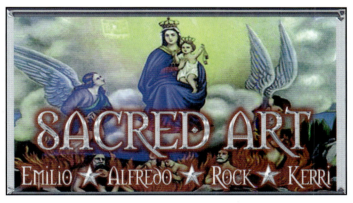

Emelio and Kerri.

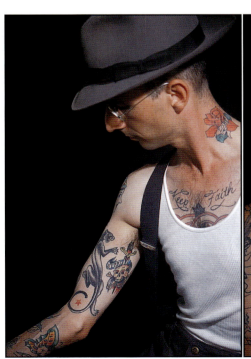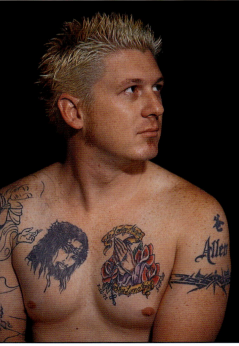

"Eric Maaske introduced me to color. I also learned by reading magazines, but tattooing is about application. If you want to learn to color, you do solid color. If you want to do black and gray, you do black and gray. It's about making as many mistakes and going as far as you can. Then you back up and see what works—what's right and what's wrong. The magazines are great, the artists in them do great work, but you can't see how they're doing it. You have to make the mistakes and discover what you're good at and what you're not so good at. I have a very good color foundation. I'm solid at what I do. The stuff I don't do, I refer to others. I won't take on any tattoo that I'm not comfortable with."

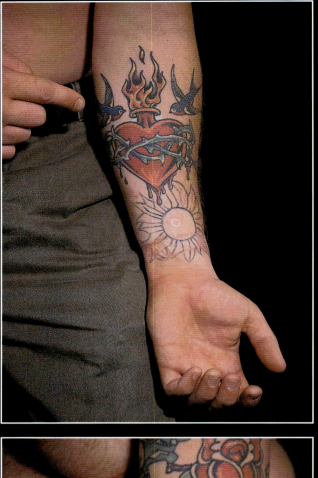
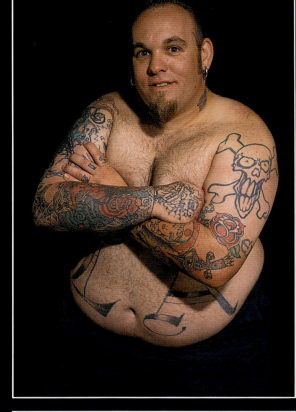
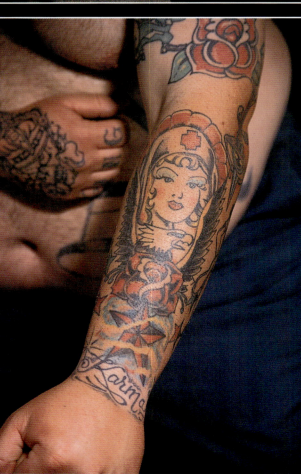
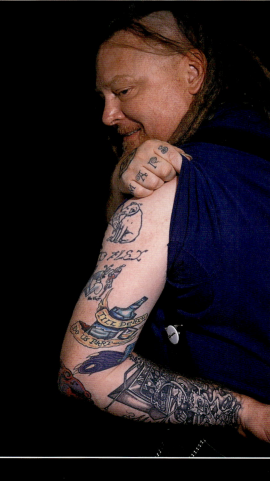

In 1995, Emelio opened Sacred Art in Gardena, the Monte Carlo for card clubbers. "There were no tattoo shops where I lived in Manhattan Beach, so I checked out the beach areas: Manhattan Beach, Hermosa Beach, Redondo Beach. None of them allowed tattooing. I headed east. The first city that allowed tattoo shops was Gardena. I got as close to the Torrance border as I could and found the nicest, cleanest corner. It just so happens El Camino College is across the street. Students generate about 60% of our business. It worked out for everybody. Within a 15-mile radius, there are no other tattoo shops. We make it a point to do quality work at a decent price. Give people more than what they ask for. It's a very diverse community: Japanese, the elite beach crowd, Hispanic, Samoans. It's great because everyone's spending their money in the same place."

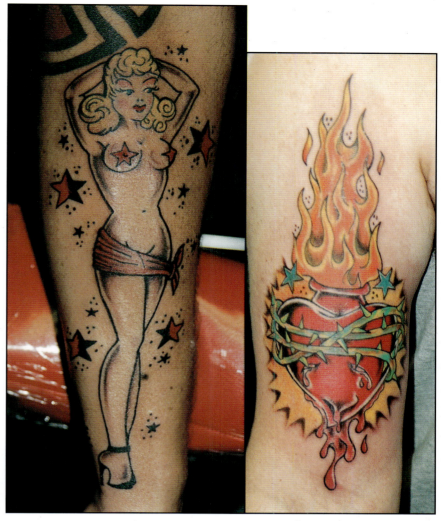

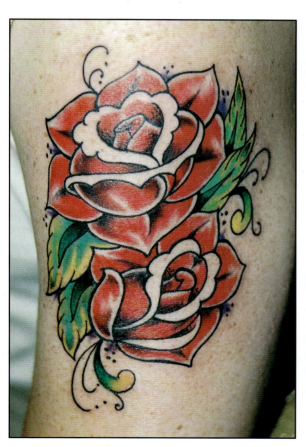

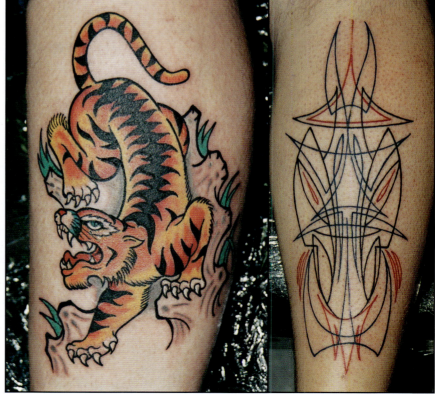

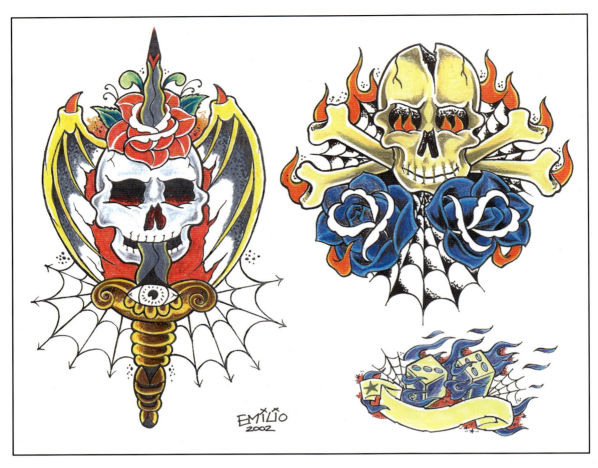

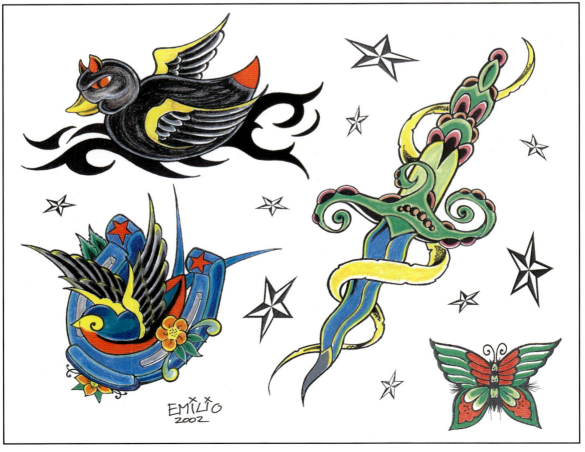

LEAP OF FAITH

While Emelio had a get-on-your-knees-and-scrub-floors apprenticeship, Kerri Hodsdon took a different route. At 21, Kerri got a free plane ticket to Los Angeles from a family friend and, with $400 in her pocket and three suitcases full of clothes, settled in Hollywood. She was interested in tattoos way before she arrived, but it wasn't until she relocated that she got heavily tattooed. She moved back to New Hampshire for an apprenticeship in 1994, but that didn't work out. One thing led to another, she returned to L.A. and happened to walk into Body Electric on Melrose.

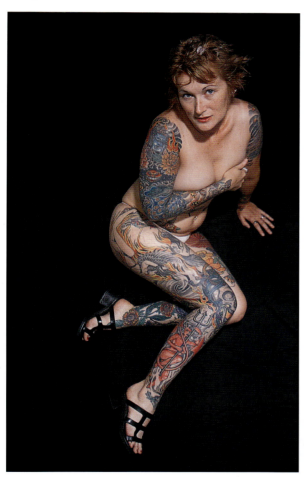

The artist herself: Kerri Hodsdon.

"I looked at the guys' books. At the time it was Pote Seyler, Jesse Tuesday, Riley Baxter and Running Bear. I was blown away. I had never seen tattooing like that. Over the next two years, I ended up getting tattooed by everyone who worked there, plus Clay Decker and Joe Vegas. And when Riley moved to Tabu, I followed him, to finish the work I'd started. That's where I met R.J. and Dottie. They referred me to Robert Benedetti and Greg James, and in 1999 I began my apprenticeship at Sunset Strip Tattoo."

THE APPRENTICESHIP

"Their apprenticeship is very formal. I was lucky enough to apprentice with both Greg and Robert. The way they did it—it was me and another guy, a longtime client of Greg's—you did lecture classes during the day with Robert, and, when Greg came in for the nightshift, he gave the practical application of the lecture, like needle making, machine building, blending pigments or whatever. It's really intensive. You've got to totally immerse yourself in it. They gave me a lot of opportunities to learn. You're welcome anytime. They don't limit the hours. Greg and Robert don't have to be there for you to be at the shop. You can ask questions of all the tattooists. You can watch people tattoo for hours, which is what I did. I was at the shop from 10 a.m. to 12 midnight, as much as I could be. I really wanted to tattoo well. It was important to me.

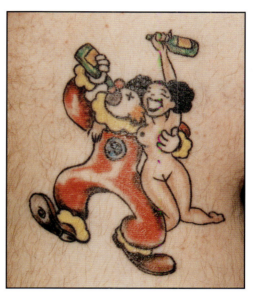

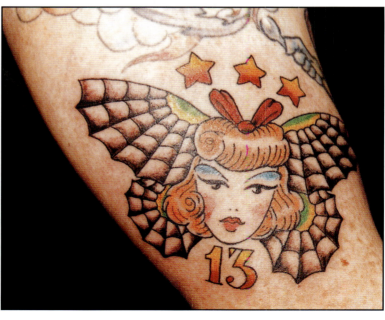

"The apprenticeship is fairly short, about eight weeks. It's not your traditional apprenticeship. Robert actually said at the beginning, 'You're paying me to be here, so don't clean the toilets. You paid for this. I don't expect you to be my slave.' Still, I always cleaned Greg's tubes, made needles for them—stuff like that. You do flash. They put up a sign that said, 'We Have Apprentices, We're Doing Free Tattoos.' You get people who are interested in that. The tattoo design has to be approved by Greg, because he does the practical end of the apprenticeship.

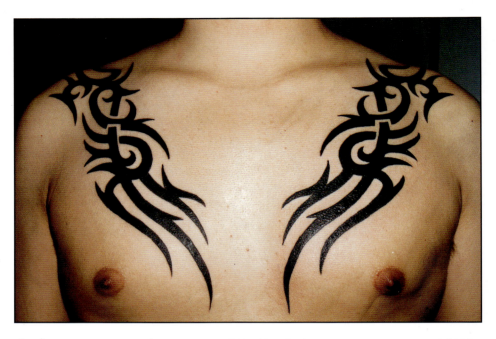

"In the beginning, the apprentice does a portion of the tattoo, the lines and a little shading. Then Greg finishes the tattoo, fixes the mistakes, goes over what went wrong and explains how to fix it next time.

"It's a very good way to learn. It gives you a head start. I know a lot of self-taught tattooists who are really great artists—it definitely helped me at the beginning. But even when you finish the apprenticeship, you're not ready to tattoo professionally."

After that, Kerri went to work at Venice Beach, because she knew they'd hire her.

"There's a lot of shops down there, and a lot of tourists. I showed like six photos of tattoos I did during my apprenticeship. I worked at Ocean Park Tattoo for three months. Then I worked on Hollywood Boulevard for about nine months at

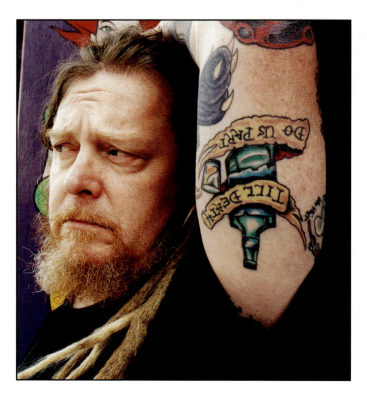

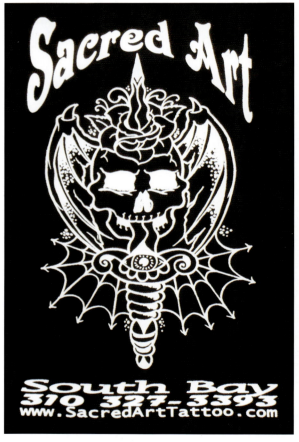

Boulevard Tattoo. Basic flash tattoos. Lots of small tattoos. Great for getting your chops up. Then I worked for the summer at Fine Line Tattoo in New Hampshire. When I came back, Dottie told me her friend Emelio needed someone at Sacred, and I ended up getting the job. I've been here a little over two years. I worked so hard to be a tattoo artist. I don't think I'd want to do anything else."

KARI & JEREMIAH BARBA
OUTER LIMITS TATTOO, ANAHEIM

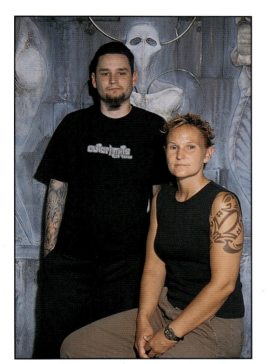

Kari and her son, Jeremiah.

Now for something completely different: a tattoo artist mom with a tattoo artist son. Enter Kari Barba and her son, Jeremiah. Off the top of my head, I can't think of another mother/son combination; certainly none with the talent and reputation of Kari and her incendiary 25-year-old.

Born in Minnesota, Kari started tattooing at 19. She learned primarily on her own, with coaching from a friend, Gil Grant. In the beginning, she mainly tattooed Gil and other local friends. The next thing, it was 1980. Kari got laid off from her job and moved to Southern California. In 1983, she opened Outer Limits in Anaheim.

"I got a call from Dave Yurkew. He told me that Cliff Raven was looking for someone to tattoo in Los Angeles. I thought, *There's no way I can work with Cliff Raven. Absolutely not, I'm just starting.* But t parked in my mind that maybe California would be the place, if I ever thought about opening a shop. The idea was planted It just took a little while to happen.

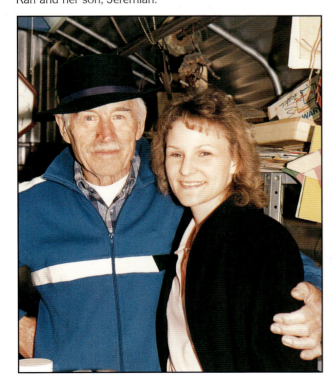

Kari with Paul Rogers, Jacksonville, Florida.

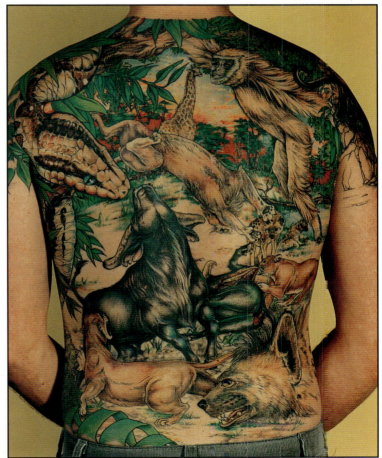

Kari Barba backpiece from the late 1980s.

Kari tattoo from 1999.

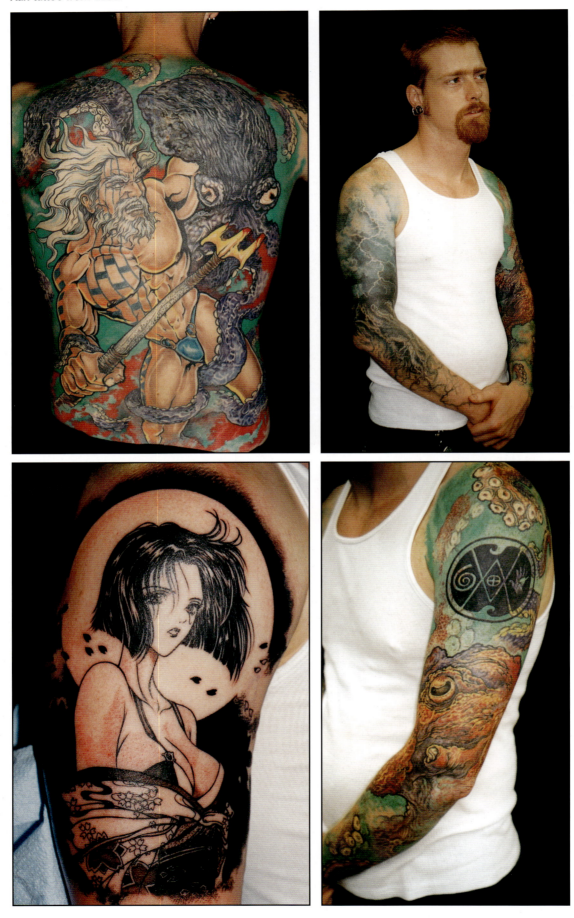

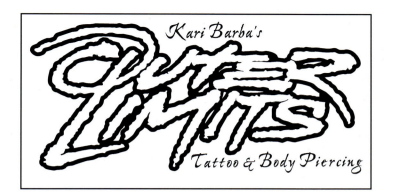

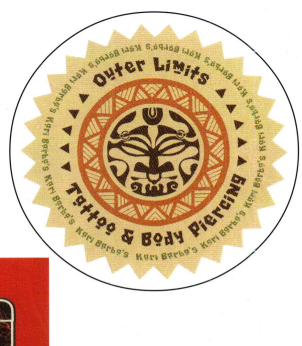

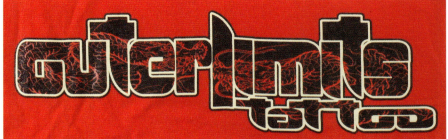

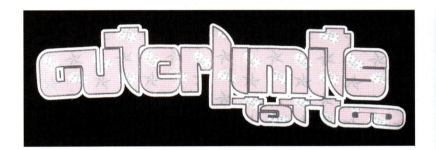

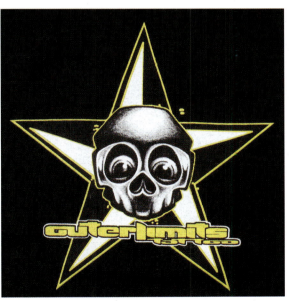

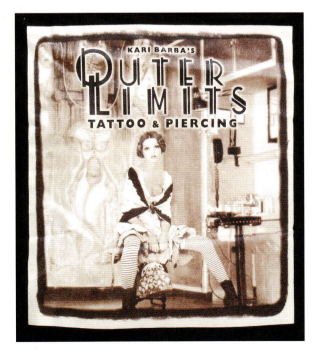

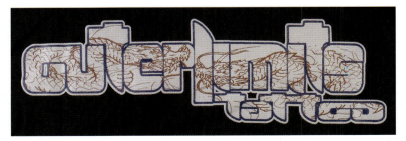

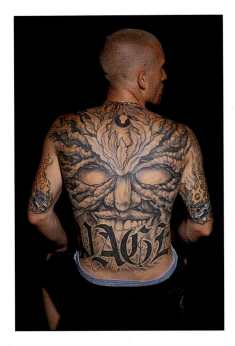

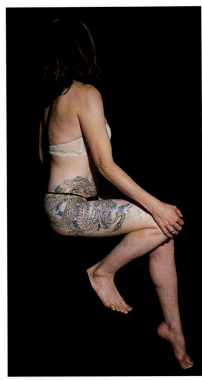

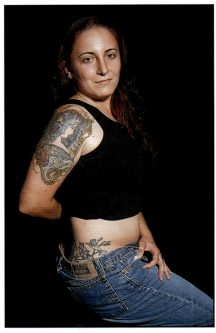

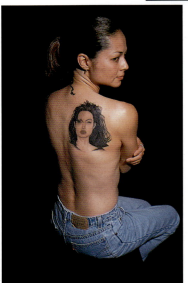

"At first, I used to hate tattoos. I didn't have too much knowledge back then. Then I started seeing more detailed tattoo art—work from people like Ed Hardy, Bob Roberts and Jack Rudy. They were doing the major work at that time. And Vyvyn Lazonga. I saw some flash she'd drawn. I was very impressed. It showed me there were different ways of tattooing from what had gone before. It sparked my interest.

"I started right off the bat doing black and gray. I didn't start color until a couple months later. I was doing mostly those little fairies and things of the time, like the Swan Song guy. That kinda stuff. Now I'm probably best known for my diversity and detailed color work. When I first started, the only person doing detailed color was Ed Hardy. Other artists were concentrating on black and gray, if it was detailed at all. That was over 20 years ago."

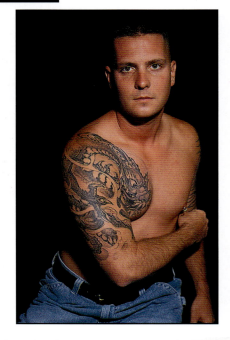

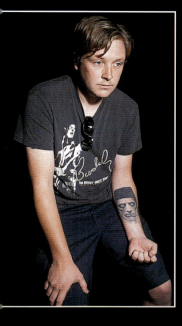

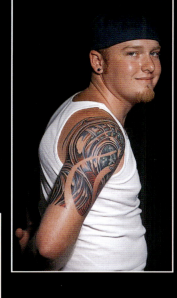

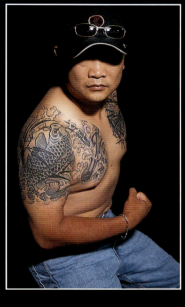

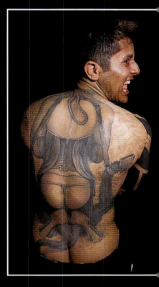

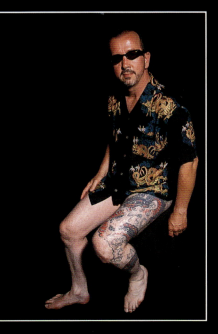

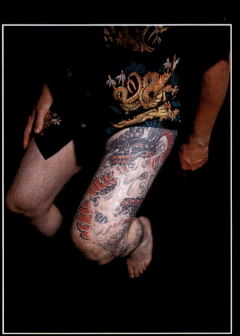

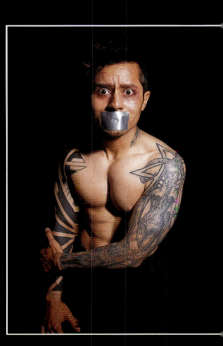

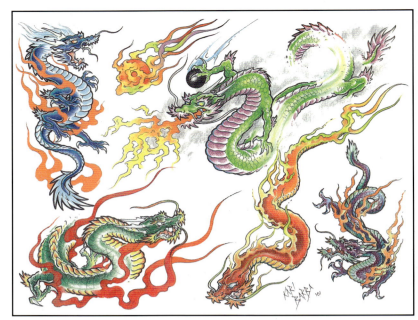

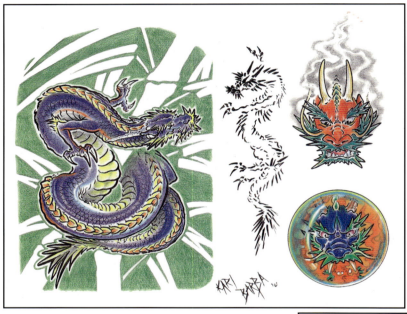

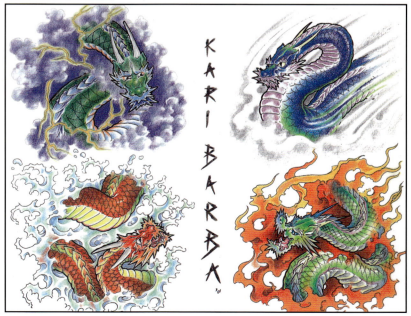

142

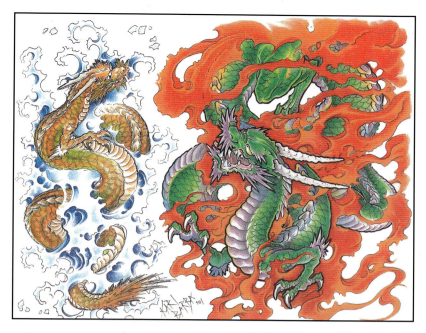

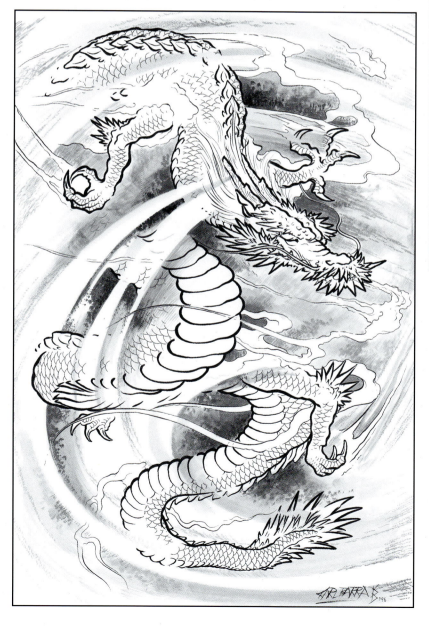

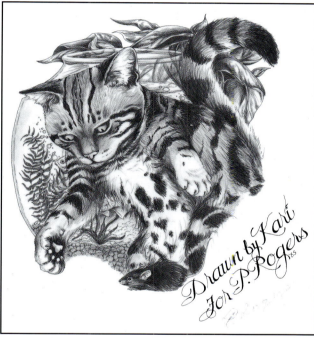

Drawn by Karl
for P. Rogers

143

THE BOY WONDER

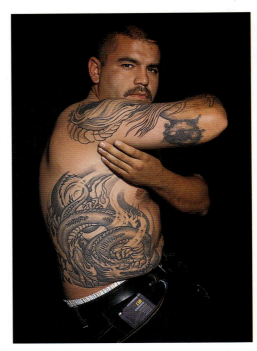

"When my son, Jeremiah, first considered tattooing, I tried to talk him out of it. It was around the time AIDS was first becoming a big thing, and hepatitis was a major fear. All the health regulations were coming into play, so I tried to push him away from it. Of course, that didn't work. He had already made a pact with tattooing. But if I had had my choice at the time, he would have gotten into law school. But ultimately it's up to him. Initially, my main concern was the health issue. There were times when he came to me and asked for some instruction, but now it's best he learns on his own. He talks with Paul Booth and Guy Aitchison quite a bit. He learns a lot from them."

Being the son of Kari Barba is not a bad entrée into the tattoo community. When you're a young man named Barba, everyone wants a peek. And what they saw, they liked. He not only has his mother's bloodlines, he's got a following of his own. Plus—and this is perhaps the most important part—he's no smart-ass kid. In a world where one-week-wonders are claiming to be "the best that ever was," Jeremiah clearly respects his teachers. And, just like his mom, Jeremiah learned tattooing very quickly.

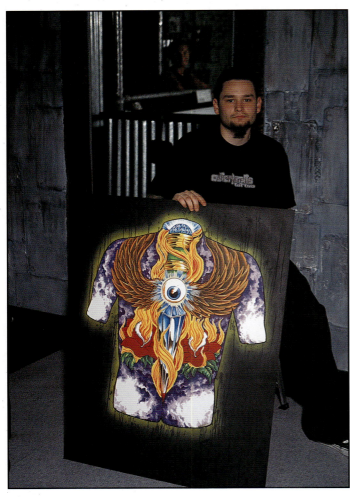

Jeremiah Barba.

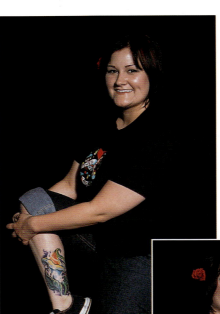

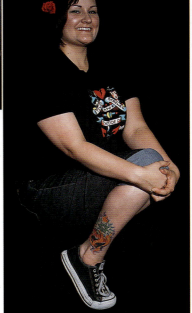

144

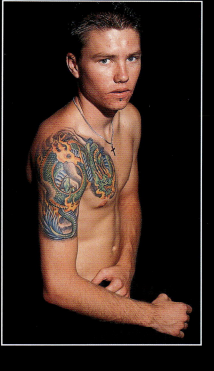
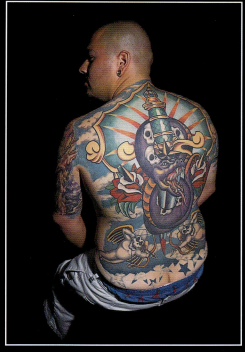
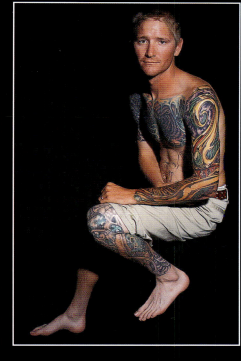
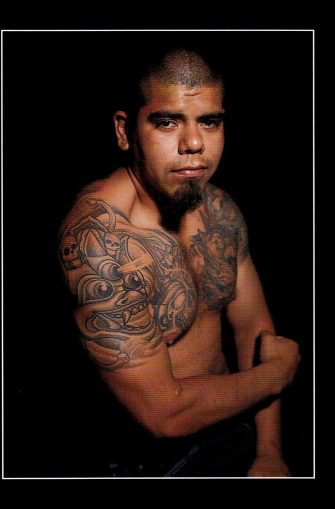
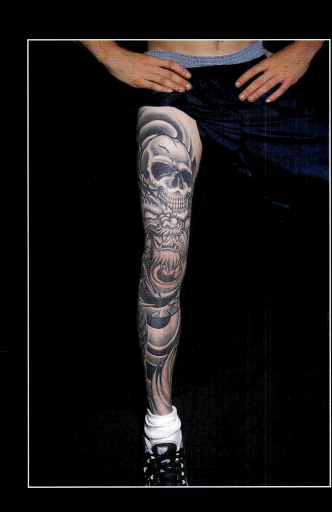

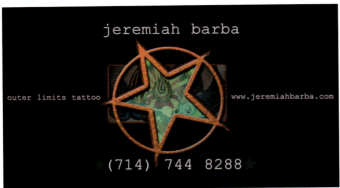

jeremiah barba

outer limits tattoo   www.jeremiahbarba.com

(714) 744 8288

"Once someone shows me something, I pick it up right away. I saw my mom draw ever since I was a little kid. A lot of my skill came from her—composition, what looks right. Recently, I've been learning about color and depth from Guy and Paul. It's funny, whenever I get tattooed by someone that good, I come home, and I want to do that style. But my mother is still my biggest influence. I'd love to work with her more. We only tattoo together on Fridays. That's not nearly enough."

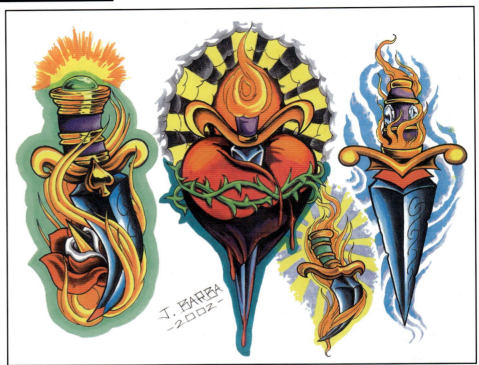

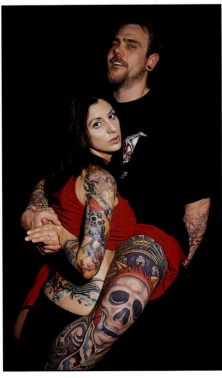

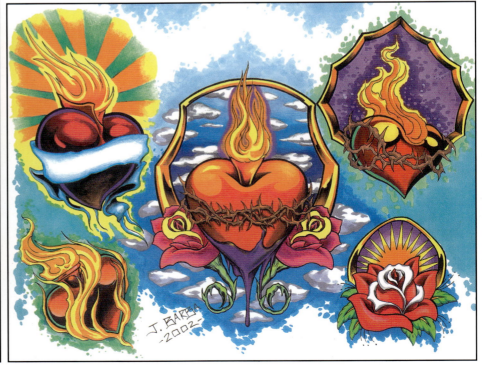

TENNESSEE DAVE JAMES
WEST COAST TATTOO, LOS ANGELES

Grand Central Market.

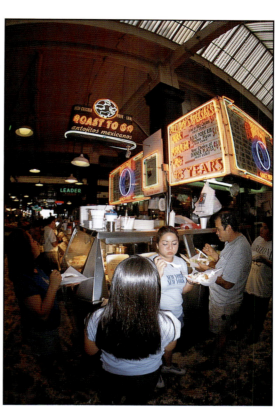

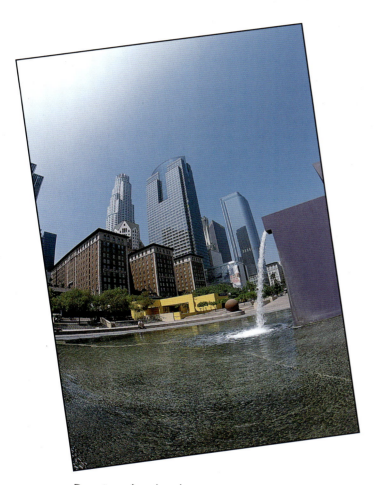

Downtown Los Angeles.

One of America's great tattoo storytellers is Tennessee Dave James. I love the guy. He's always up and running. Nestled in the heart of downtown, his shop, West Coast Tattoo, has lots of foot traffic, but it's mostly pitiful panhandlers, foggy-headed drunks and ne'er-do-well grifters. Amid this chaos, Dave is headman at one of L.A.'s oldest and most authentic tattoo shops. No thick carpeting here. No waiting area with gushy couches and smiling shop girls. This is West Coast Tattoo, L.A.'s eye-of-the-hurricane street shop.

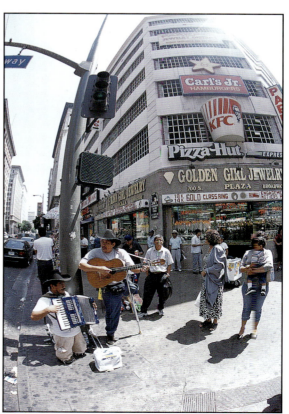

Street corner minstrels.

When they made Tennessee Dave, they broke the mold. The older brother of Greg James, Tennessee Dave never runs out of stories. For many, his column, *The Wit and Wisdom of Tennessee Dave*, is a priceless connection to the way it used to be, before there were shops on every corner, back in the days of the Pike. It's been a long, colorful road for Tennessee Dave, and I for one wish there were more like him. Tough, kick-'em-in-the-ass funny, and a heart of gold.

"I first got hooked on tattoos in Chicago in 1956. That's when I got my first tattoo from Alexander, the 'World's Greatest Freehand Artist.' I remember the first time me and my buddy went down. We didn't have any tattoos, and we didn't have any I.D. We weren't old enough. So Alexander says, 'If you already had a tattoo on your arm that I could cover up or something, we'd make an exception for ya.' So my friend and I went home and got a bottle of India ink, scratched a little something on our arms, let it heal up, went back down there and said, 'Hey, can you cover this up?' He said, 'Sure, sit down,' and from then on, that was it. It was all the way. I was hooked."

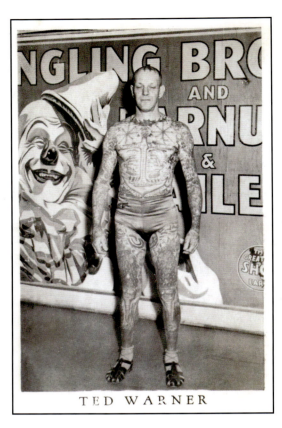

Ted Warner pitch card, 1950s.
Photo courtesy of Tattoo Archive.

TED WARNER

LONG-TERM EMPLOYMENT

"I didn't actually start tattooing until 1963, when I came out here to Los Angeles. I was working for a wheel and trailer place out on Slauson and Western. Continental Wheel & Trailer. Drove a truck and a forklift. I used to hang around the tattoo shop after work. West Coast Tattoo, the same shop we're in now, but back when it was at 507½ South Main. Just around the corner. It was hang around, hang around, hang around. I used to go for coffee for Sailor Ted Warner. After a while, the owner of the shop, Captain Jim Malonson and his wife—it was coming on summertime—they were getting ready to take off for the home they owned in Mexico. So Teddy's telling them, 'You know, I'm here alone. I need some help here.' So Jim says, 'Why don't you grab that knucklehead and teach him how?' That's how it came about.

"At that time we were the only tattoo shop in the whole city. There were no tattooers in the San Fernando Valley. There was nothing in Hollywood. There was nothing in Venice. The nearest other place to us was Long Beach, and from there it was Oceanside, going south. Going north, the nearest shop was probably Oakland or San Francisco. There was nothing in between. We were it.

"Eighty percent of the work we used to get in those days was guys from the San Fernando Valley. Bikers, we got a lot of bikers. Plus the military and a lot of Hispan-ics. Right here on the corner where the welfare hotel is—that was condemned at one time—but the mezzanine floor was the USO. Every Friday afternoon you'd see the buses coming from Camp Pendleton with the Marines. They'd drop them right off at the corner, and we'd have them until Sunday night when the buses came to pick them up. We had them all weekend. We'd stay open 24 hours. I had the 11-to-nine shift. I'd tattoo Marines, one after the other. During the week, we got the hard-core Valley guys that didn't want to wait until Saturday. On weekends, all the Valley people would go to the Pike, because they'd take their families. They'd go for the rides and the amusements."

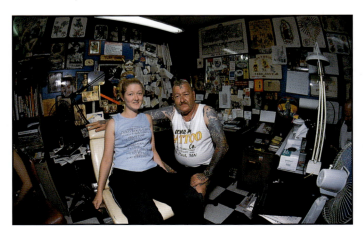

Tennessee Dave and his daughter Frances.

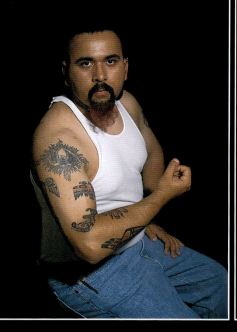
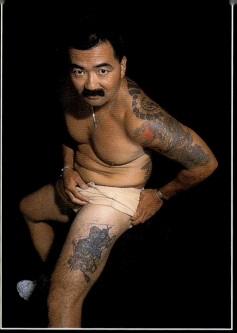
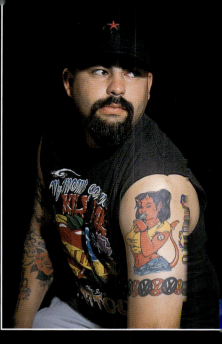
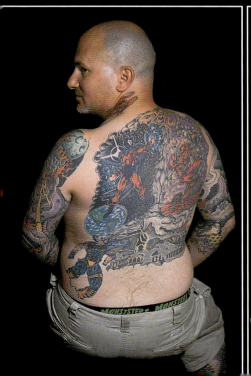
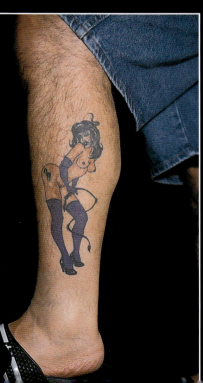
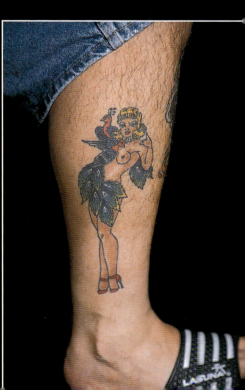

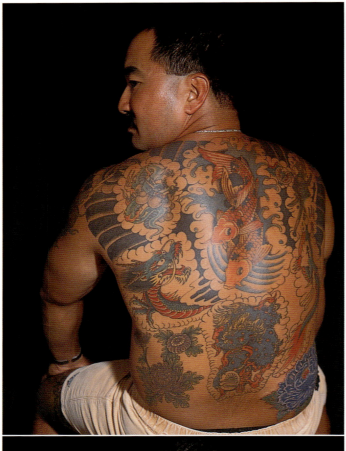

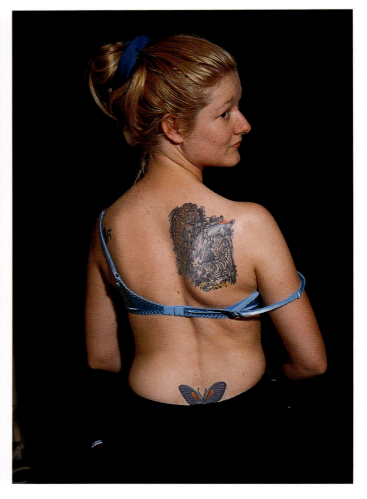

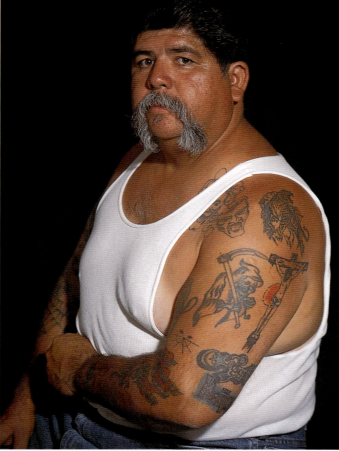

THE PIKE

"The Pike was the center of tattooing in Southern California during that time. That and San Diego. I used to work at the Pike. I was still working for Captain Jim, because he owned a shop down there. He went partners with Fred Thornton. I worked in that shop. I used to work at the Pike on weekends. I'd work during the week in downtown L.A. and, on Fridays I'd pick up my brother Greg, and we'd go down at 4 o'clock and work the shift on Friday, Saturday and Sunday.

"At the Pike, there was Bert Grimm's shop at 22 Chestnut. And up on a little side street off Chestnut was Fred Thornton. The next one up from Bert Grimm's was Lee Roy Minugh's. Owen Jensen worked in there. What a nice old gentleman he was. I used to go in there at night when there wasn't any business and just talk to him. When I first started going down there, that was it. It didn't expand until Captain Jim hooked up Fred Thornton with Al Orsini. They had closed down the old 40 [Four Oh] Cafe—it was actually a bar, not a cafe. Jim said, 'You know, that would make a great shop.' It was huge. So we did. It still had the bar in there, so instead of a rail, we just cut the bar in half, right down the middle, and left it standing there. That was a great place to work. We didn't have a name for it. It was just Tattoo Shop.

"Up until then, the only people working down there were the people working at Bert's. There was Don Nolan, Tom Yeomans, Rio de Janeiro. That was Lou Louis's son. His real name was Lou de Janeiro. He named his son Rio. It wasn't a stage name. Rio de Janiero. That's who was working there—Bob Shaw, Larry Shaw, and Bobby Shaw, when he wasn't in jail, and Tom Yeomans, Hong Kong Tom, and Don Nolan. They worked at Bert's. Fred Thornton worked alone, he never had anyone working with him. And then Lee Roy and Owen Jensen worked together. Lee Roy worked days, and Owen worked nights."

GETTING BETTER

"Nowadays, I like the fact that everyone is more open. In the '60s, if I wanted to go down the street and visit Bob Shaw, Jim would say, 'Stay out of there. Don't go near that guy.' That was the attitude all the way up through the '20s, '30s, '40s and '50s. They didn't trust one another. They figured you were coming down to steal business from them. Steal a secret from them. That's the way it was. Everybody knows everybody by their first name now. The ink and dyes are much better and so is the technique. In the '50s and '60s, you couldn't get a portrait of somebody's face done. And you couldn't get anyone to take the time either. In those days you

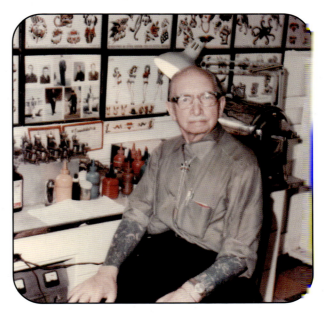

Owen Jensen, Long Beach, California, 1960s.
Photo courtesy of Tattoo Archive.

had a shop full of people who wanted to get tattoos. If somebody came in and said, 'I want an eagle fighting a dragon,' it was, 'Go down the street. We don't want to fuck with that. We're busy doing roses and hearts for five and ten bucks. We don't want to spend time doing that.' It wasn't going to put money in their pockets. That's why Sailor Jerry's pinups had their hands behind their heads—so he didn't have to do fingers."

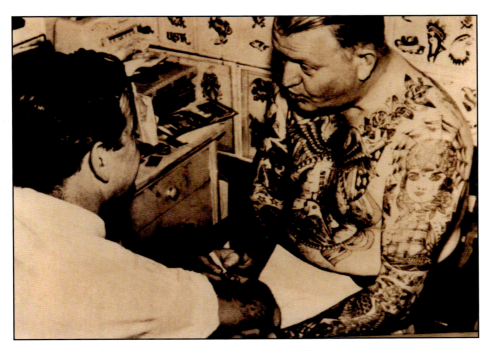

Lee Roy Minugh tattooing in Long Beach, California, 1960s.
Photo courtesy of Tattoo Archive.

JOHN SALETRA &
COLIN LAROCQUE
TABU TATTOO, MAR VISTA

John Saletra spent his formative years in Youngstown, Ohio. When he hit 20, John decided to see the world and moved to New Orleans. He stayed there for about four years. Then down to Miami for two, before he found the place he'd been searching for as manager of Tabu Tattoo in Mar Vista. "It's a comfortable happiness," says John who enjoys the big, roomy shop owned by R.J. Musolf and his wife, Dottie. "I love the environment and the people that work around this area," adds John. "I'm here to stay."

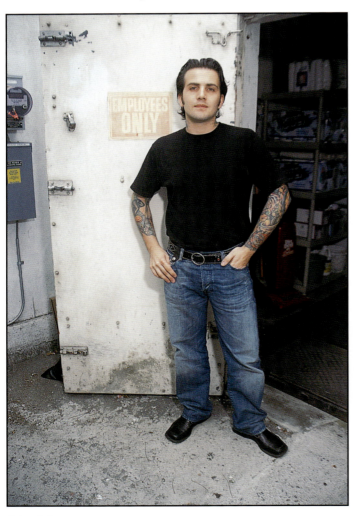

John Saletra.

It's not difficult to see why John was chosen to run the shop for two of the friendliest people in the business. Tattooing for eight years, John's warmth and humility go a long way in carrying on Tabu's tradition of being one of the most inviting, attractive shops in town. Handling the responsibility of running a shop and dealing with people seems to come naturally to John. Observing him at several conventions, he hangs with the class.

"I was always into tattoos," John explained. "When I was young, I used to draw on my arms. I came from a family where tattoos were really taboo. Something just clicked with tattoos. I got one, and I enjoyed it. It helped remind me of a point of time in my life. Kind of like taking a picture and carrying it with me always. I always had a love of drawing, but it grew as time progressed and turned into an obsession. It became a lifestyle for me, more than anything else.

"Much of what I learned came from traveling. I met people who taught me the difference between right and wrong in tattooing. Each tattoo requires specific elements. Certain images in Japanese tattooing, for example, need to be expressed using specific colors. And when they're not there, it's not correct, and you give someone a tattoo that is meaningless. That's why I study constantly, ever since I became really serious, about five years ago. There where people that made me realize the effort and research necessary to tattoo properly. Real, true art needs to have the proper research and history behind it. That's one of the reasons I like to travel, to collect books and go to conventions. I'm so lucky to be in Los Angeles. Greg James, Bob Roberts, Mark Mahoney—those three are such incredible tattoo artists. I'm so lucky to have Greg James working on my back. I'm so lucky to sit down with him and talk about tattooing. It's a fulfilling experience. There's no doubt about it, the wealth of information available in Los Angeles is simply amazing."

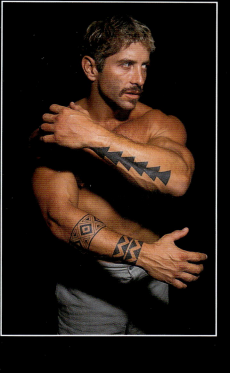
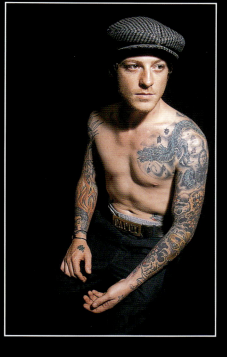
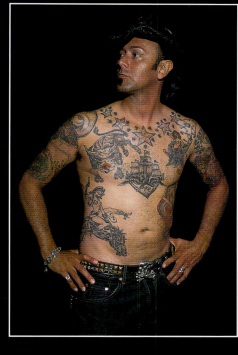
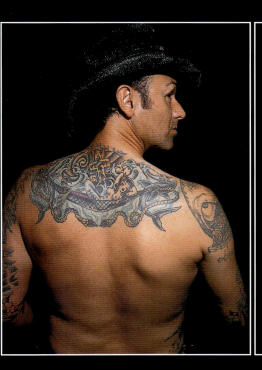
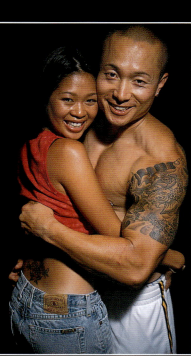
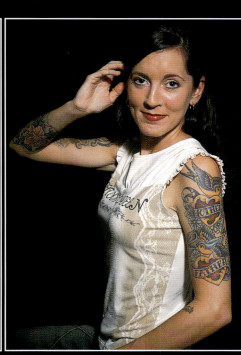

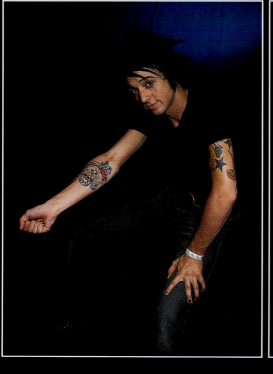
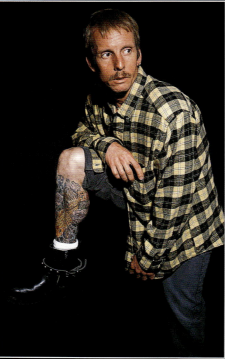
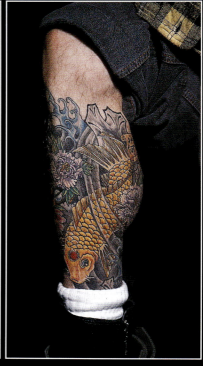

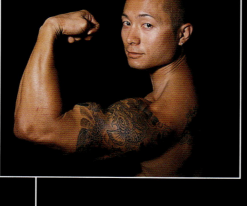

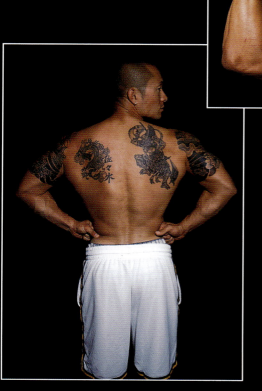

The lads and Dottie in front of the Venice Boulevard shop.

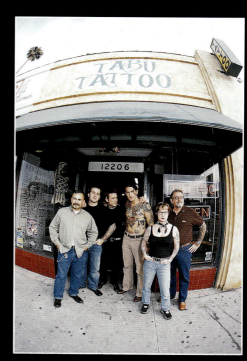

154

BORN IN A SUITCASE

Originally from Toronto, Ontario, Colin LaRocque's parents were in a Top-40 lounge band. When they started getting gigs in New York State and east of the Mississippi, young Colin joined them on the road. They finally ended up in North Carolina. It was around Thanksgiving, and everyone was wearing shorts and T-shirts. According to Colin, "The weather was nice, so the family decided to park it."

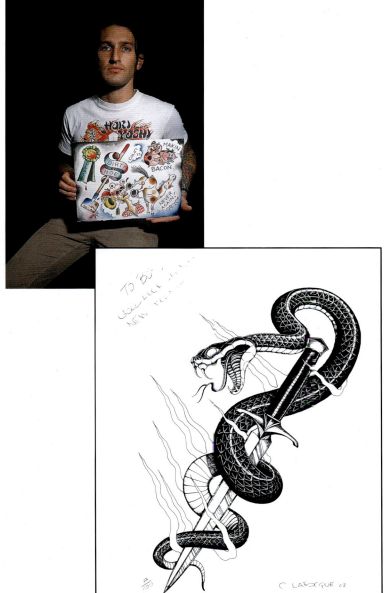

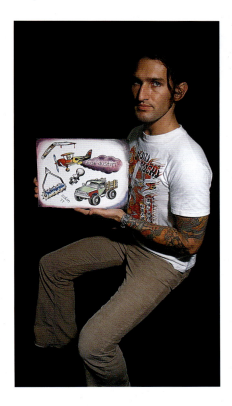

Colin LaRocque shows off his farm flash.

Colin was about 16 or 17, into carving things from wood. It was 1992. Colin was playing drums and ended up living in a band house where everyone had tattoos but him. He asked where they got theirs, and they took him down to John Rainey at Alternative Arts in Charlotte. "We ended up getting to know each other a little bit, and he offered to apprentice me. I'd just watch him work. He taught me the bare minimum, what to do, and I took it from there. Then I came out to California to play drums with a guy from North Carolina. Juan Puente put in a good word for me—he said he knew a shop that needed some help—and, luckily, I got a job at Tabu."

This is all fine and good, but what I really wanted to find out about was Colin's farm flash.

"I was just going to do one sheet of it, really, as a joke. And then I thought, *Maybe I need to market this like I'm really serious. See what people say*. It seems like everyone started to take it seriously. I've already done some pieces off the set, and customers are really digging it. I don't think there's anything out there like it."

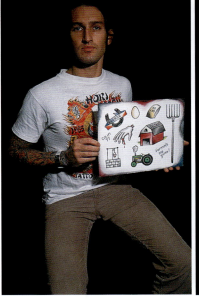

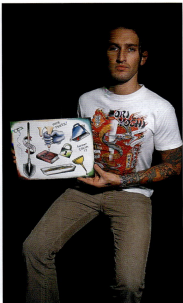

RILEY BAXTER
BODY ELECTRIC, HOLLYWOOD

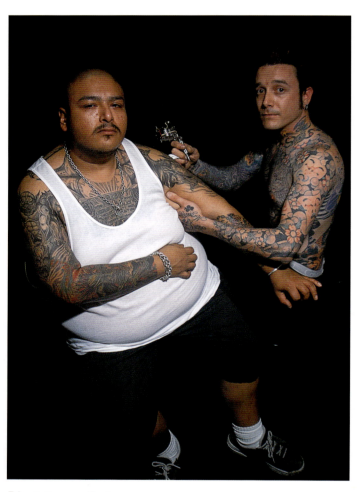

Riley tattoos a client.

My son Riley Baxter gave me my first tattoo. A *koi* fish on my left shoulder. He was working with his brother Jesse at Body Electric at the time. I got the tattoo for two reasons: One, I liked the aesthetics of the *koi* fish, and, two, I wanted to show support for Riley's chosen trade. Up until then, Riley was quite nervous when I'd walk in on him putting designs on friends at a tattoo party. No matter how strongly I affirmed my approval, Riley sweated bullets. Until the *koi* fish.

Along with the personal empowerment I felt with finally having a tattoo, I noticed a great deal of positive feedback from Riley's circle of friends when they discovered he had tattooed his very own father. There was a definite buzz whenever I entered a room. I was accepted

in Riley's inner circle. I recall attending Riley's performance with Snair. After introducing myself as Riley's father, the bartenders bought all my drinks. I was the *tattooed dad*—an immediate and respected celebrity.

I have a foggy understanding of the burgeoning of Riley's career as a tattoo artist, but I thought it a good idea to set the record straight.

THE BLUE BLOB

"The first people who got me interested in tattoos were friends with political slogans tattooed on their arms. That's when I first went, 'Whoa!' I'd seen tattoos on older people in public and old friends of yours. As a kid, I noticed a blue blob that was maybe an eagle, but I didn't really think about it. The first time I really said, 'Look at that tattoo, can I see that?' was on my friend Greg Eisenburg; it was a dead skeleton army dude. He was hunched over a foxhole-type machine gun, like he'd been shot. And it said, WAR CANNOT BE WON. I thought, *That's cool!* I was in high school. I didn't have a car yet. I was 15.

"Whenever I picked classes in school, if it was an art class like drawing or painting I'd definitely take it, but if they didn't have any more space or I'd taken that class a bunch of times already, I'd take industrial art. That way I learned graphic layout and whatever. I'd be up all night drawing on the arm of my friend Matt's leather jacket with Sharpies. Or I'd stretch a T-shirt over an art board. Not even put a tracing underneath it, just eyeball different punk slogans. And I'd wear them next day to school. And all my friends were like, 'Where did you get that shirt?' I ended up drawing shirts and running into friends at clubs. I asked my friend Greg, 'Where did you get your tattoo?' and he said, 'Spotlight Tattoo on Melrose.' So, on my 16th birthday, first thing, I drove down and got my first tattoo from Bob Roberts."

The way Riley got tattoo equipment was by hanging out at Venice Bob's. He went into the shop in Santa Monica sporting his leopard-spots hair with spikes. Riley told them, "My little sister got tattooed here, and I really want to tattoo. I don't have any gear, and I don't want to do it the wrong way." He showed them some artwork he'd done, T-shirts and such, and, duly impressed, they got Riley some equipment. Then they let him do a couple walk-ins, because the other guy that worked there didn't show up. The next thing 17-year-old Riley knew, they fired the other guy. Riley stayed a couple years. That was 1986 or '87.

DROP ON BY

"I met Kevin Brady at Venice Bob's. Kevin and I decided to join forces and tattoo in motel rooms, do tattoo parties at my friends' houses, like that. We'd all be drinking beer and tattooing so we could live. After about five or six months, I ended up going into Sunset Strip Tattoo. Greg James had seen my work and told a friend of mine, 'You should bring Riley by some time.' I'd been in Sunset before, but it was very intimidating. Here I was, returning years later. Robert and Greg were there, Little Mike Messina and Rick Rockwood. It was a Friday night, and that's how I met all of them. That must have been September 1987. Then next year I started at point A with those guys. I was there until 1992. That's when I went to Las Vegas for about six months.

"Then I came back to help Rick Rockwood open his shop in Studio City. It was perfect timing. I didn't have to be there 24 hours a day and was recording the first Killing Machine record. After that, Pote Seyler had just opened Body Electric with Running Bear. After about a year, my brother Jesse Tuesday and Kevin Quinn went there to work. So I rented this killer warehouse-style, five-car garage, where I lived and tattooed for two years. It was right off of Melrose on Spaulding Street, about six city blocks from Body Electric. Actually a couple tattoo-magazine covers were tattooed out of my house. Then Kevin Quinn left Body Electric, and I was there about five years. The day Jesse left Body Electric to go to work for Eddy Deutsche at 222 San Francisco, I went to work at Tabu for Bob and Dottie. It was 1998.

"I love Bob and Dot. They're the nicest people in the world. But now I want to do a bunch of traveling. I do more than just tattooing. I'm writing songs and playing bass with a couple of bands. I'm kind of like a hobbyist, like my mother. I do a lot of different things. I'm currently ripping up my rugs, because I just found out there's a hardwood floor under our carpet. I'm so stoked.'

Always on the move, Riley left Tabu and is back at Body Electric.

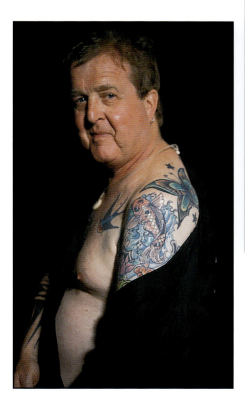

The famous *koi* fish.

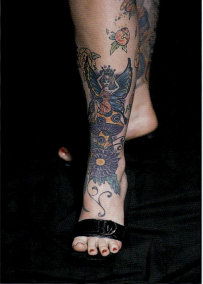

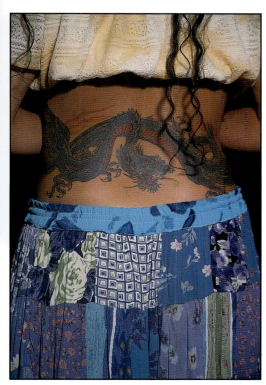

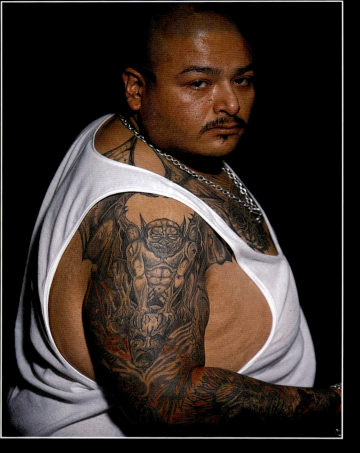
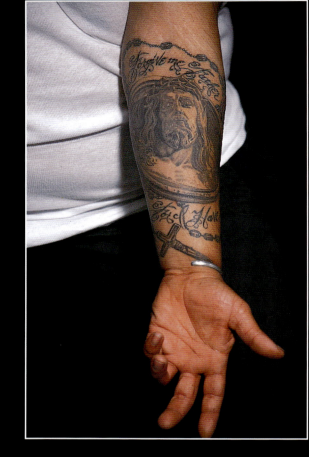
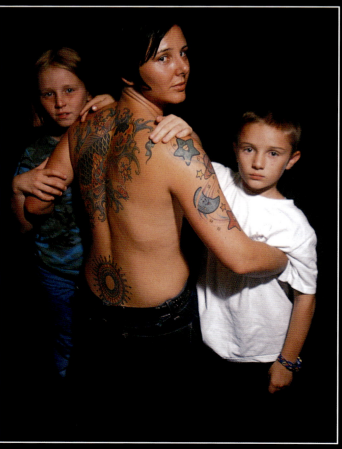
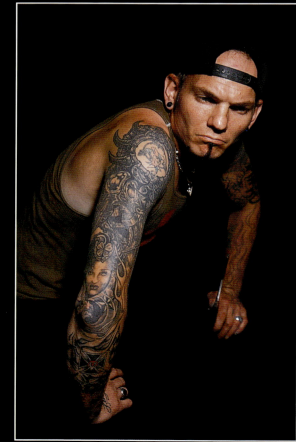

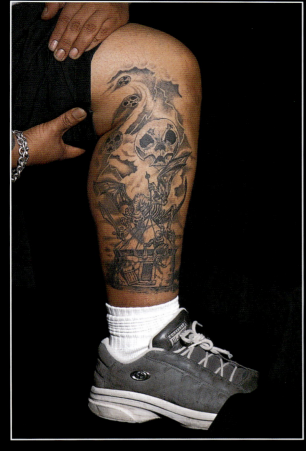

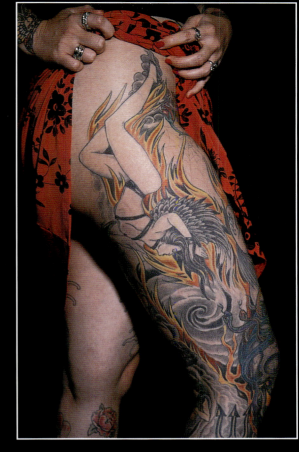

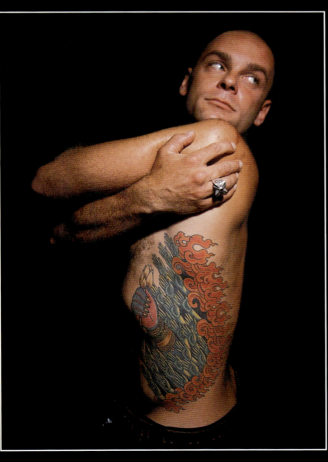

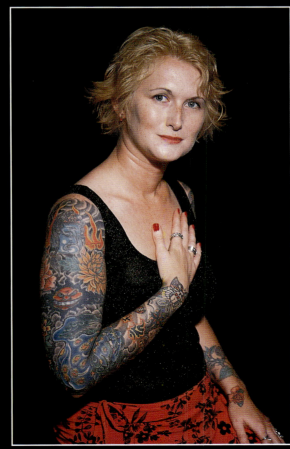

SHAWN WARCOT
EMPIRE TATTOO, RIALTO

When I tell people I drove out to visit a shop on Route 66 in Rialto, most of them ask, "Where's that?" Even native Californians! Well, for your information, Rialto is just off the 10, a short burro ride east of San Bernardino, in an area we in Southern California lovingly refer to as the Inland Empire. And on a cloudless August afternoon, it's hotter than hinges.

I used to go to school just east of San Berdoo at the University of Redlands. Back then, they used to roll up the sidewalks at dusk. Times change, and Shawn Warcot has a corner on tattooing in the Inland Empire. He is not only a talented artist, but a charismatic entrepreneur with a slew of shops.

"I'm partners with Mike Tryke. We have shops in Rialto, Riverside and Redlands. I'm an Air Force brat. My father retired and located in Riverside, and I never left. I got tired of moving around. SoCal seemed like a good place to be. I was 15. I pretty much grew up in the Inland Empire. Tattooing is something I always wanted to do. The first time around, it was 1978, I was 18, painting custom cars and bikes, you name it, from the time I was 16, all the way up to 27. I came in to get my first tattoo from Mike, and we hit it off. He took a look at my portfolio and decided to train me. I'm 41 now."

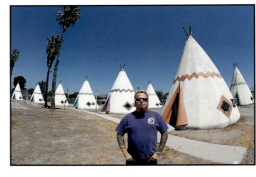
Shawn at the trailer park.

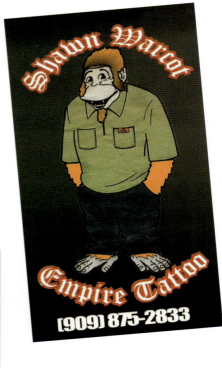

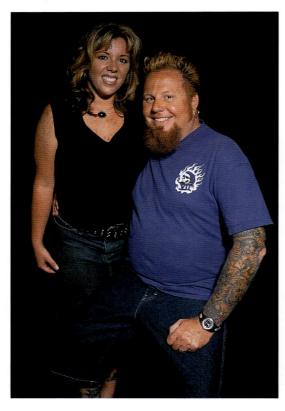
Shawn and his wife, Amy.

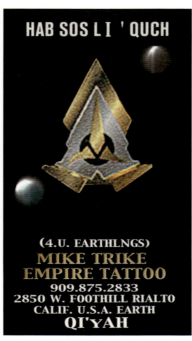

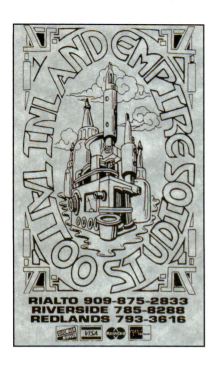

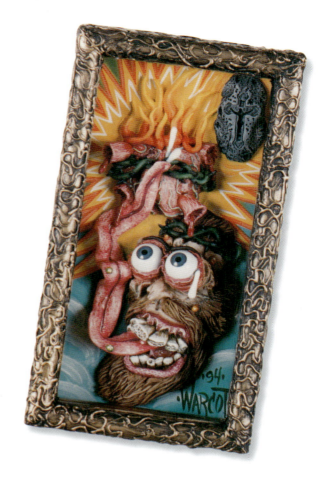

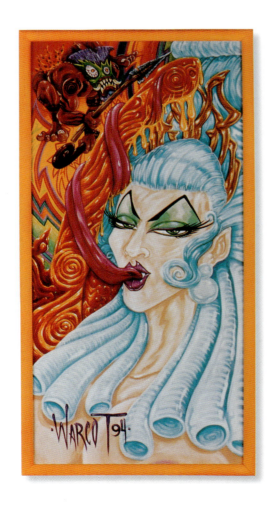

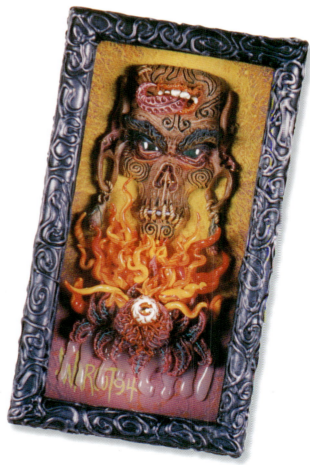

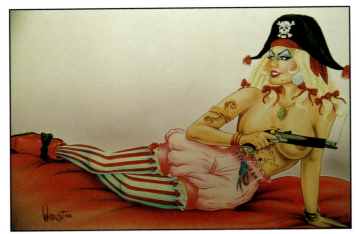

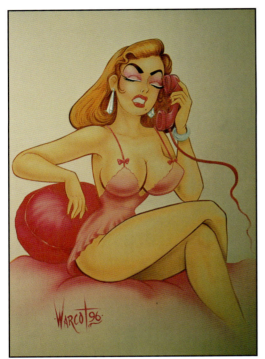

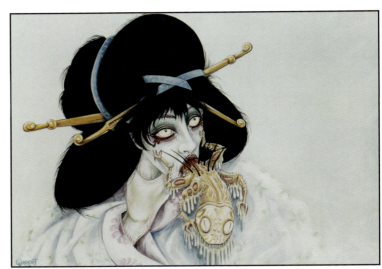

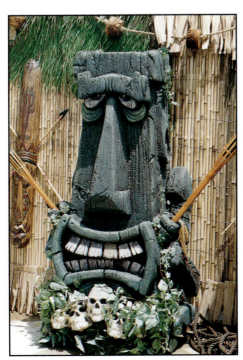

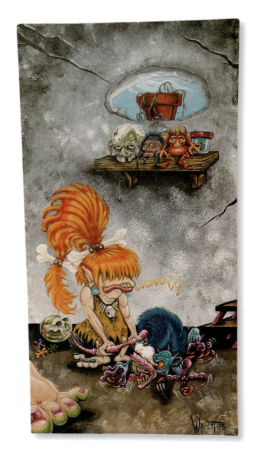

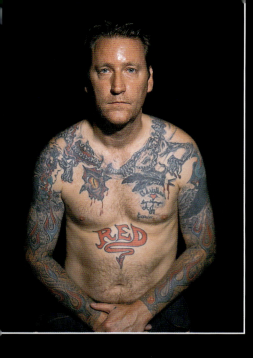
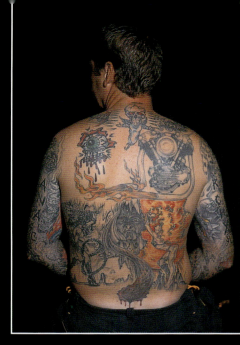
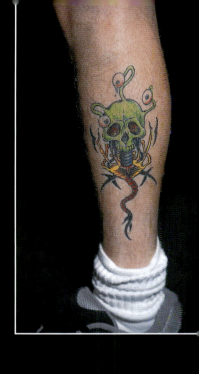
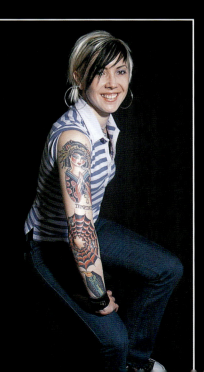
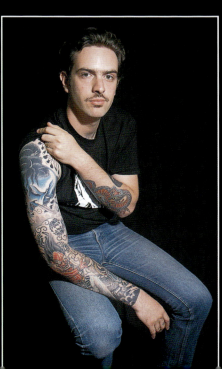
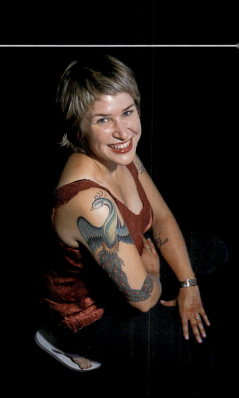

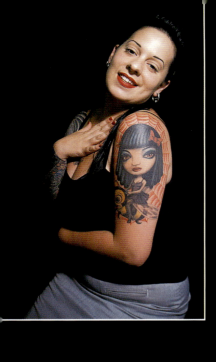
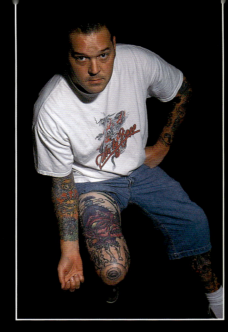
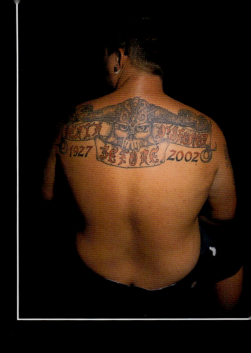
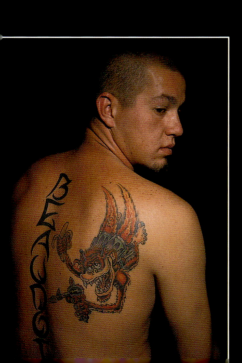
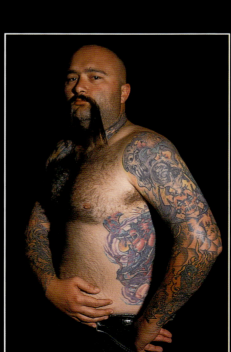
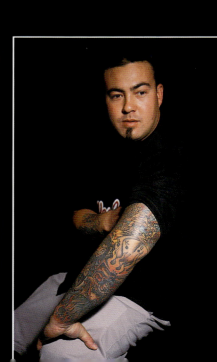

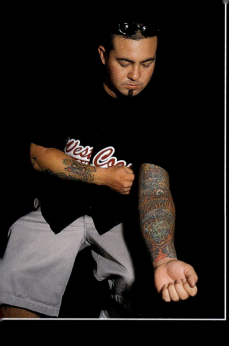
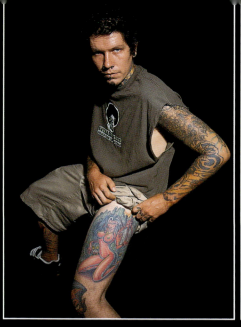
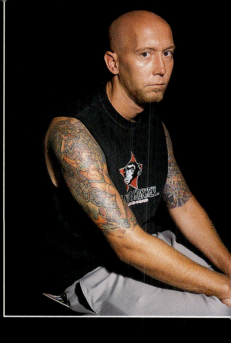
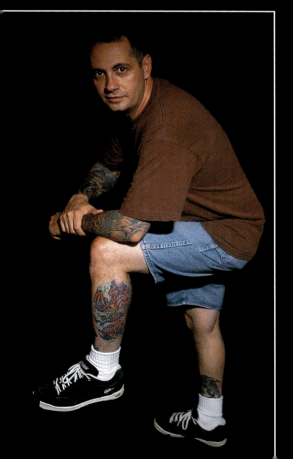
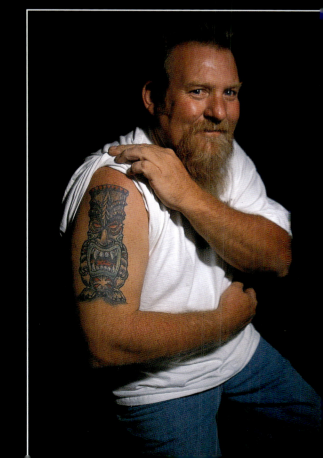

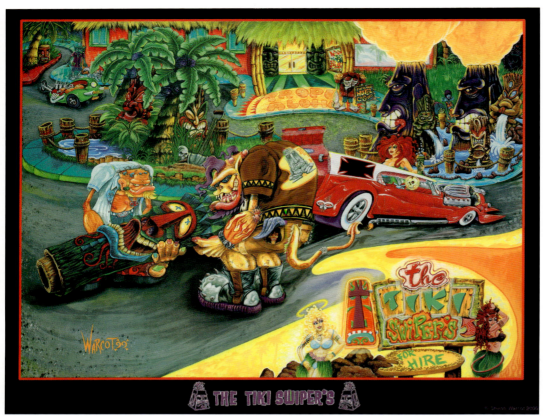

THANKS TO GRANDPA

"My grandfather had some girl's name tattooed on his arm from the Korean War, but that's it. No one else in my family has tattoos. This guy Jesse next door was a biker, a custom painter. He was the influence when I was a kid. Bob Roberts, Fip Buchanan are the two artists I admire the most. Now we're the best-kept secret in the Inland Empire. We've been here 15 years, and business has stayed fairly steady, probably due to the quality of the artists. We always try to have the most credible artists, and, when new talent crops up, we make an effort to recruit them over to us.

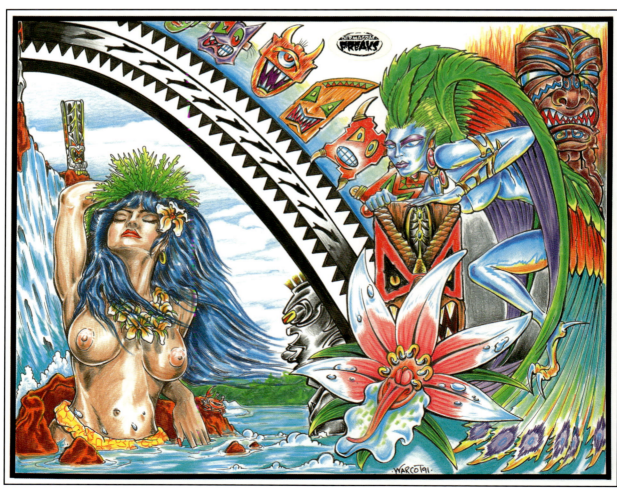

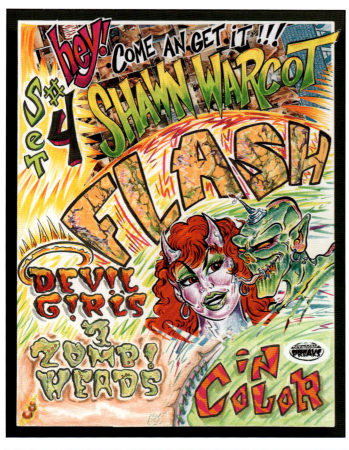

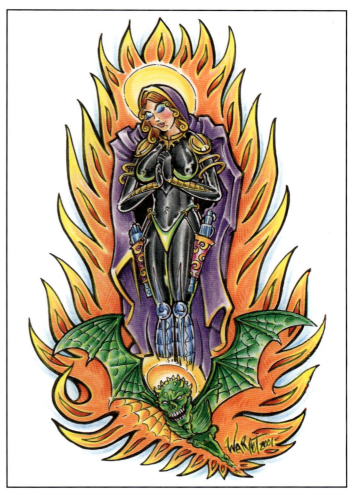

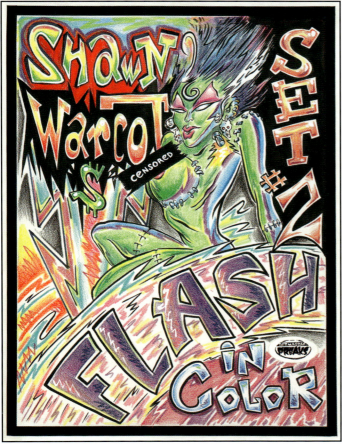

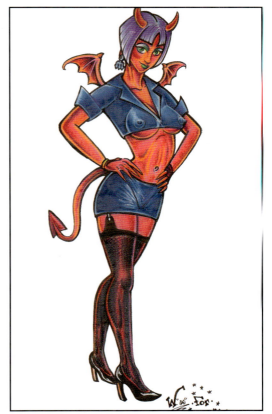

"We're only the an hour away from L.A. True, there's probably more wizards done here than in Los Angeles, but if we introduce our clients to new ideas, they usually get it. We rotate our flash, and all of our guys are custom artists, so we're not too far behind the big city. Maybe a fraction."

Being the most easterly stop on my itinerary, it was a pleasure to see a few remnants of old California. Not before-it-was-a-state old, but back-when-I-was-little old. It made me recall when Route 66 featured those amusing Burma Shave signs. One line of the rhyme was posted every quarter mile or so, and we'd all shout the words in unison as they appeared up ahead. A phrase at a time, we'd yell it out. Including a big, loud "Burma Shave!" at the end.

Don't lose your head
To gain a minute
You need your head
Your brains are in it
Burma-Shave

The wolf who longs
To roam and prowl
Should shave before
He starts to howl
Burma-Shave

Santa's whiskers
Need no trimmin'
He kisses kids
And not the wimmin
Burma-Shave

Altho we've sold
Six million others
We still can't sell
Those coughdrop brothers
Burma-Shave

This, of course, was a reference to Smith Bros. cough drops logo and its beard-wearing namesakes, Trade and Mark.

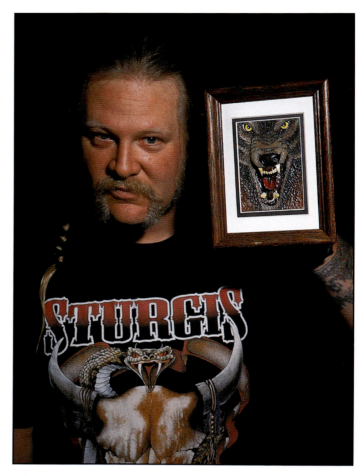

Mike Tryke shows off his leatherwork.

After I packed up the cameras, Mike showed me some of his amazing leather carving, and Shawn walked me over to the concrete teepees. Yeah, I remember those from when I was a kid. Those were the days. And what a joy it was to return to the scene of my boyhood memories, to stand in front of the famous Wigwam Motel.

VISIT 23
JUAN PUENTE
SHAMROCK SOCIAL CLUB, HOLLYWOOD

When I heard a new tattoo studio was opening on Sunset Boulevard in Hollywood, I went, "Oh, no. Just what we need; another bleedin' tattoo shop." If memory serves me right, wasn't there a hubbub when Tattoo Mania opened only five minutes down the road from Sunset Strip Tattoo? Over time, that worked fine, as did Sunset relocating a sneeze away from Purple Panther at Sunset and Stanley. Everyone seems to be getting along swimmingly. But another shop just a brick's throw from Tattoo Mania? Heaven help us.

But what at the outset seemed folly, turned out brilliantly. The difference, of course, is that under the leadership of its owner and guiding light, Mark Mahoney, Shamrock Social club immediately became one of Southern California's two great power shops (Bob Robert's Spotlight being the other). Amazing! Quite a testimony to the status, within the industry of its founder, Mr. Mark Mahoney.

One statistic I find quite telling is the fact that Shamrock's Juan Puente was also part of 222 San Francisco when *that* shop, at the end of the 1990s, was one of the two pinnacle shops in San Francisco, along with Ed Hardy's Tattoo City. I think it's more than coincidence.

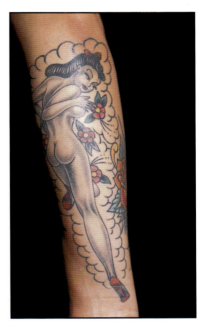

Juan Puente tattoo.

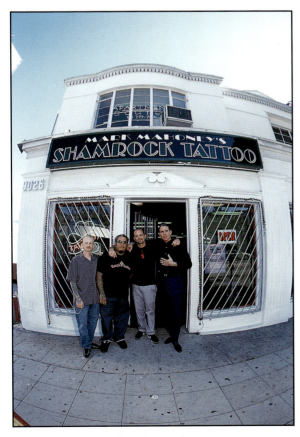

The Shamrock Social Club.

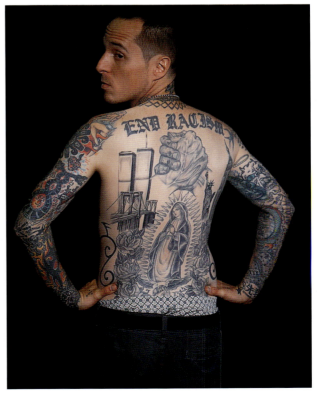

Juan Puente tattoo.

ORANGE COUNTY TRANSPLANT

I got to know Juan Puente when he worked with my son, Jesse Tuesday, at Eddy Deutsche's 222 San Francisco. Eddy closed down the shop a couple years ago, and Jesse moved to Las Vegas. I kind of lost track of Juan in the shuffle. Originally from Orange County, Southern California is Juan Puente's home. In high school he did the usual flyers, leather jackets and such. At first, he wasn't into tattoos, until when he was 21, on a whim, he got inked by Joe Satterwhite. That changed everything. Juan had friends who were tattooing, like Corey Miller, and one thing led to another. In the last 12 years, Juan has worked at Avalon in San Diego, 222, of course, then Eric Maaske's Classic Tattoo in Fullerton. Now Shamrock.

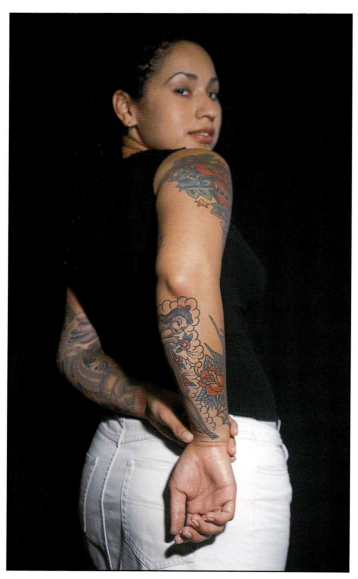

Juan Puente tattoo.

MARK MAHONEY

When I arrived at the shop, Mark was bent over an intricate Celtic back panel. He got his signals crossed about bringing people for me to shoot. "I was supposed to do what?" said Mark, as I loaded my cameras with film. Hey, he's a busy guy, and, worse yet, since Mark, the leader of this prestigious pack, doesn't keep photos, his 411 was handled by Juan.

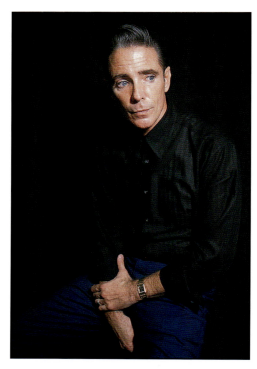

Gentleman Mark Mahoney.

"Mark came from the Tattooland school of black and gray," says Juan. "Guys like Dick Warsocki, Creeper, Jack Rudy, Freddy Negrete, Mark Mahoney, Mike Brown, Danny Romo—those are the guys that started it all. You don't see any of it now, but Greg James did ridiculous black and gray even before then. Mark's work was around. Back in the '80s, it was amazing to see his tattoos on people. To this day, he's famous for what he does and how he does it. Even so, Mark works as hard if not harder than anyone at Shamrock. If I leave at two or three in the morning, he leaves at four or six. That says a lot for someone who's been doing it 20-something years, you know what I mean? He's not afraid to do what the people ask. He has his favorite style, but he's not above doing this and that. Plain and simple: People want to get tattooed by Mark Mahoney.

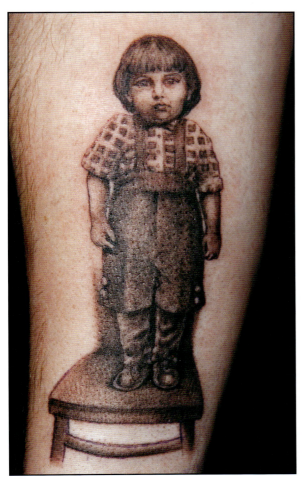

Mark Mahoney tattoo.

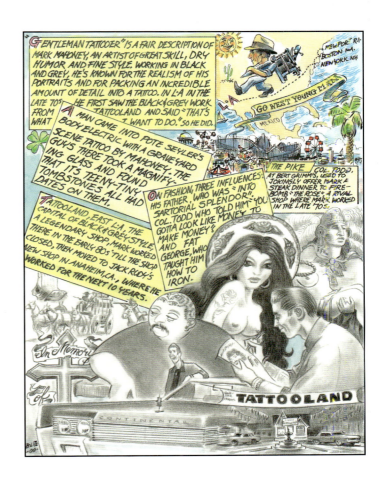

"Mark used to work up the street at Tattoo Mania, when it was owned by Gill "the Drill" Montie. Gill set a precedent of how a Hollywood tattoo shop is run—the late hours. There were no shops open late (open from noon to three a.m.) before Tattoo Mania. It was unheard of. Some shops were open from 12 to 12, doing shifts, but Gill really made the space. If you were in Hollywood and going to do your thing, be up late, that was the place to get tattooed. Gill established that. Now, if you want a tattoo at three, four, five in the morning, get a tattoo, have breakfast—it's not common in L.A., but, hey, they do it here at Shamrock."

SMALL PAUL

I know just about everyone at Shamrock—Cris Garver, Duel, Cisco—but there were a couple new faces. I was surprised to see Danny Dringenberg. I knew Danny when he ran a shop in Pasadena. It was good to hear him brag about his beautiful daughter Teresa's fledgling modeling career.

Another new face was Paul Stottler. The fact is, I wasn't familiar with that name and couldn't put together in my mind where he fit on the tattoo family tree. And when he told me, "I used to work for Jack Rudy," I didn't know what to make of it. In all the time I've known Jack, he never once mentioned a Paul Stottler.

Then he told me, "I used to go by Small Paul."

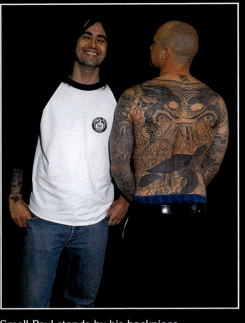

Small Paul stands by his backpiece.

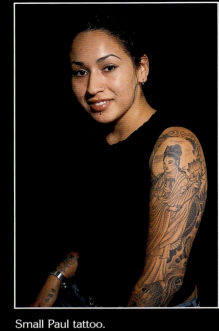

Small Paul tattoo.

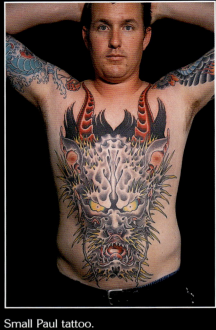

Small Paul tattoo.

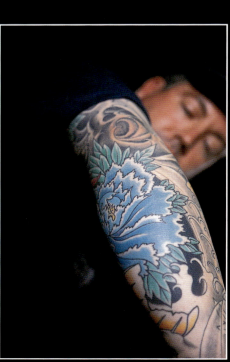

Small Paul tattoo.

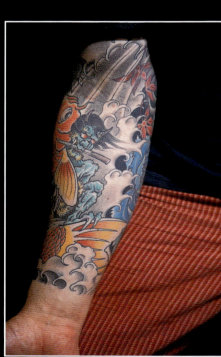

Small Paul tattoo.

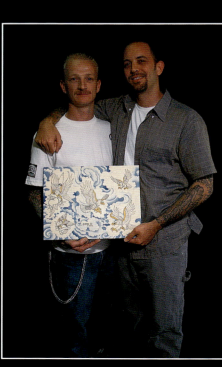

Danny Dringenberg (l.) and Chris Garver.

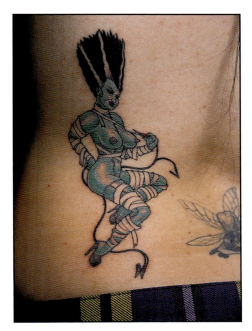

Chris Garver tattoo.

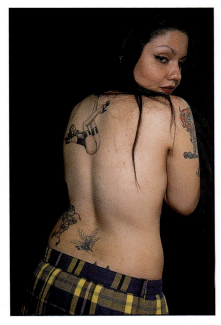

Chris Garver tattoo.

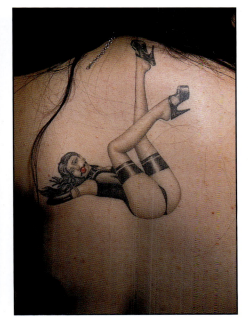

Chris Garver tattoo.

"Oh," I said. "So you're Small Paul. You I've heard about!"

Then, after I apologized about 500 times, Small Paul told me about himself and the lifestyle that has kept him under the radar the last 14 years.

Paul Stottler began his tattoo career in Arizona under Jim Watson. Then, in '93, Paul hired on at Jack Rudy's Tattooland. From then on, he used the name Paul Small. He gives Greg James credit for getting the gig with Jack. It seems Creeper was looking for people. Everyone was gone, and they needed a new crew.

"They just hired Jeff Harp, and Greg called and gave the good word. I showed Creeper my book, and he gave me a schedule. It all happened rather fast. Greg has been a great influence on my career. He's one of the rare people in this business that is genuinely nice. He's always inspired me and been supportive. He's always had time to talk to me. Every time I come out with flash, he and his brother always buy the first set."

Paul, Mark and Juan go way back. It was natural that he end up at Shamrock. But mostly Paul's at True Tattoo, where he partners with Clay Decker.

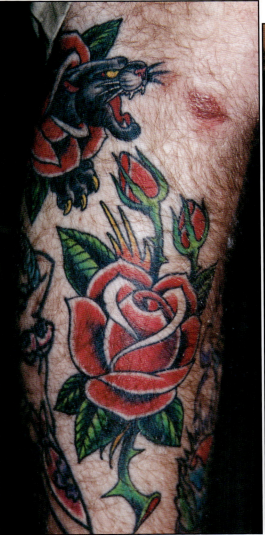

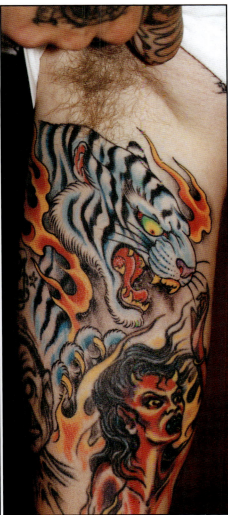

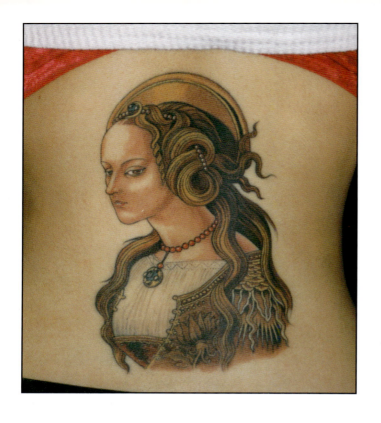

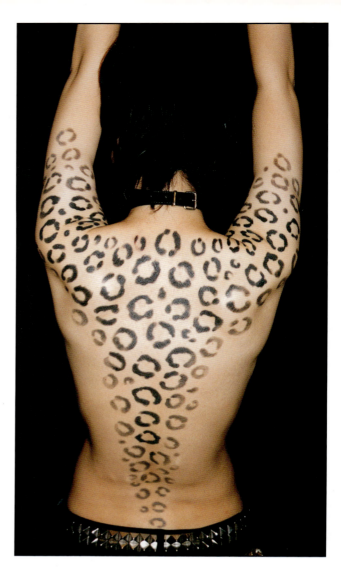

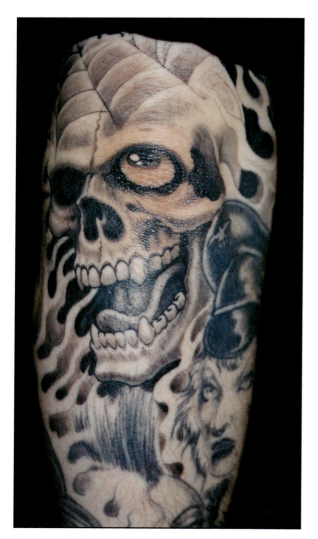

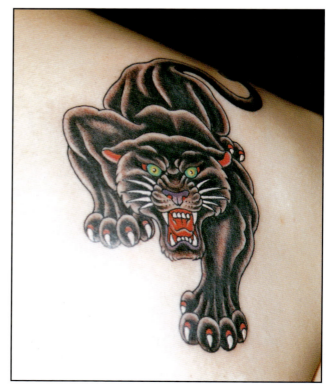

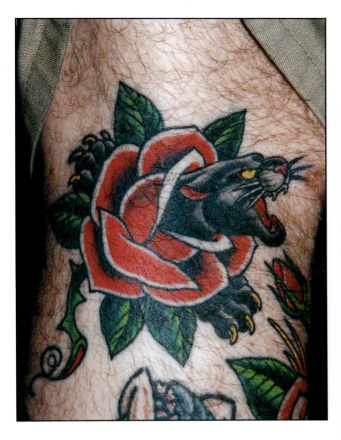

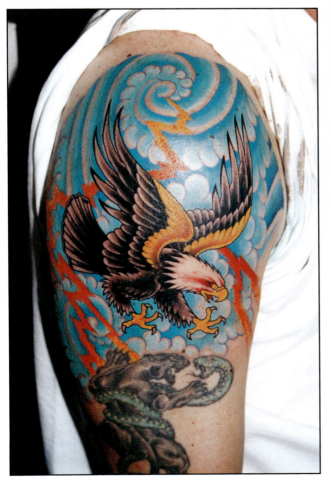

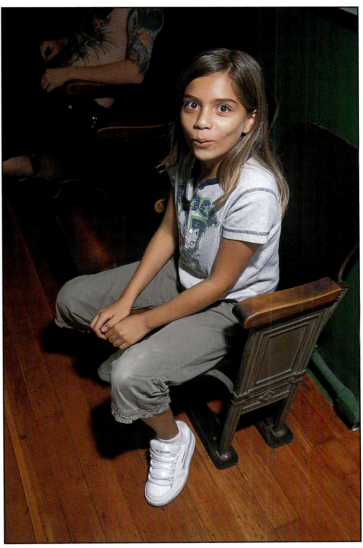

Danny's daughter, Teresa.

"I work at Shamrock one day a week. It gets me out of the house. I enjoy the opportunity to tattoo with friends I don't usually work with. To me, the tattoo scene is my close friends."

RORI KEATING
TATTOO GALLERY
HILLCREST, SAN DIEGO

I first met Rori Keating at Leo Zulueta's Black Wave, before Leo relocated to Michigan. Rori was always comfortable to talk to, without any tinge of arrogance attached to working for the legendary Leo. I also spent some time with Rori in Samoa, at both the first and second tattoo conventions in 1999 and 2001.

Born and raised in Massachusetts, Rori Keating moved back to Ireland with his family when he was 12. The first member of his family to be born outside of Ireland, Rori spent his high school years on the Emerald Isle and returned for college in the U.S. His drawings gravitated toward the abstract.

"I became interested in tattooing rather late. I hear a lot of customers tell me they were interested in tattoos, but don't know why and don't know where. I understand them perfectly, because I was the same way. And then I saw the book *Modern Primitives* with Leo Zulueta's stuff in it. I thought, *Oh, there's this style other than pictures*. Picture tattoos are cool, but it's not what was working for me. It never occurred to me that you could tattoo abstract designs. Then I started getting books and going to the library, but there wasn't very much out there.

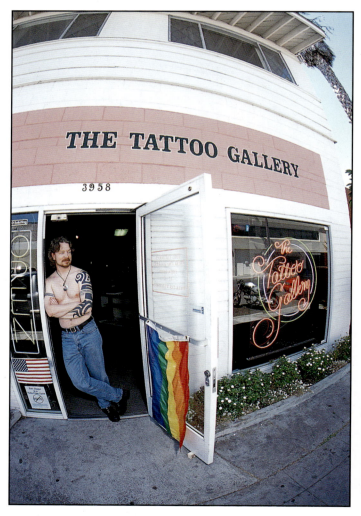

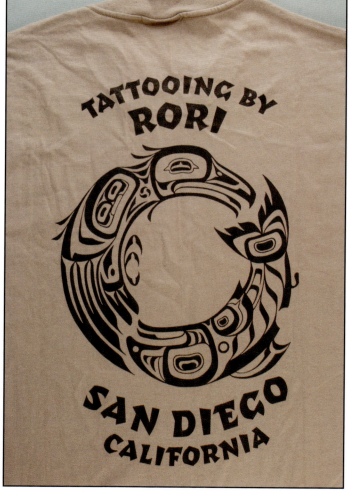

Rori Keating at the door of his Hillcrest shop.

"I worked in the theatre for years. I didn't end up getting my first tattoo until I was 28—a band of triangles around my ankle. That was before I knew there were Hawaiian tattoos made up of triangles. People told me, 'Oh, you have a Hawaiian tattoo.' I didn't know I had a Hawaiian tattoo. It was a design I just came up with out of my head. It was made up of straight lines, and I didn't realize that tattoo artists generally don't like to lay down straight lines. I like tattooing straight lines and geometric designs. Most people don't."

LESSONS FROM LEO

Rori started tattooing when he was 33. He had gotten a couple of armbands from Petelo Sulu'ape at a convention in San Diego. And then he got lucky and apprenticed with Leo. Both Rori and his wife were big fans of Leo's designs in the magazines and decided they'd both get big backpieces. "She actually committed before I did," says Rori. "We went to his shop, Black Wave, and met him. I learned from Leo, along with other art-ists in the shop: Pedro Belugo, Vincent Weiner and Adrian Gallegos, who's at Body Electric now. But basically it was all about learning Leo's style. All in all, I was at Black Wave two and a half years."

Shortly thereafter, Leo sold the shop and moved to Michigan.

TRIBAL TATTOOS

"We use the word *tribal* to describe the designs I do, but depending on how you want to argue it, if it's a contemporary design, it's not tribal. The word *tribal* describes the look, but they're not actually from a culture that uses tattoos as part of its tradition. To me, tribal is simply a visual description. What I do is study the designs from different cultures, and learn as much as I can about it to be sure I don't screw something up and create a design that is actively bad. I think it's Ed Hardy that said, 'In this country, the tattoos that are really tribal are biker tattoos and military tattoos, because the drive behind them is tribal.'

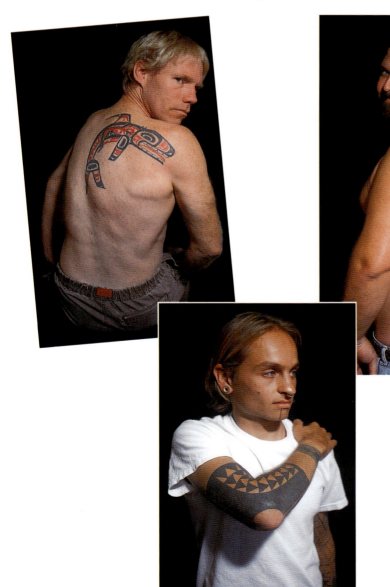

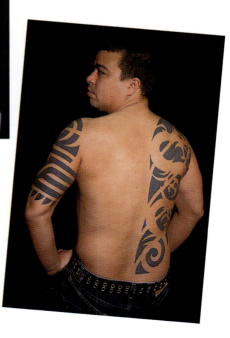

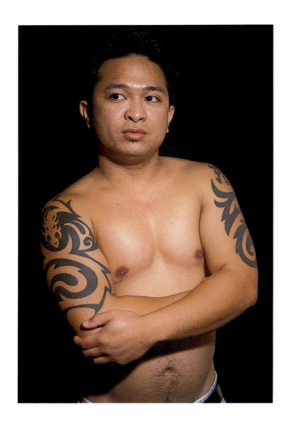

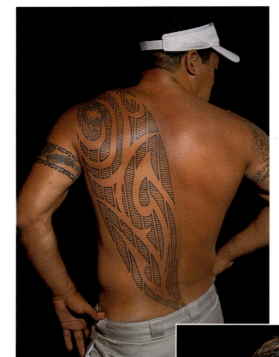

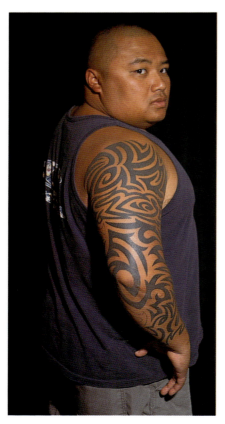

"As for Leo, his first set of flash that came out in 1991 you see bootlegged in every tattoo shop in the world. When people think tribal, they think specifically of his designs, the whole flowing style he developed based on Borneo designs. He told me that two things that influenced him were Borneo tattoos and hot-rod flames. I'm sure there were lots of other influences, but the concept of tribal designs didn't exist in the minds of Westerners before Leo came along. He opened up people to a whole other way of tattooing. He's very careful never to copy anything directly. He may use a Hawaiian design, for example, as an inspiration, but if you showed it to a Hawaiian they would say it's not a traditional design. He actively attempts not to copy anything. That's the same standard I follow."

BABY RAY
SPOTLIGHT TATTOO, HOLLYWOOD

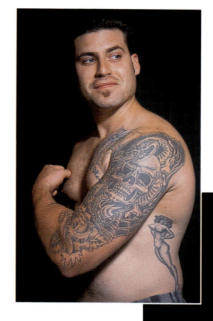

Baby Ray was under his car, covered with grease, when I first visited Bob Robert's Spotlight Tattoo. I'd set a hard and fast rule: If someone isn't at a shop when I do a shoot, I pass. Like with the Pacific Northwest book. When I came to town, if a shop was closed, I couldn't get them on the phone, or they were out to lunch, I had to move on. I had to, to stay on a strict time schedule. Consequently, some excellent artists got left out.

Ray called during that shoot at Bob's. I didn't like saying no.

But rules are made to be broken, and a book on Southern California isn't complete without Baby Ray.

Funny, but aside from his custom cars, the main thing I remember about Baby Ray was the time in Tokyo at the first-ever Tokyo Tattoo Convention. I can still see it as if it were yesterday: about 30 of us parading through the Tokyo subway station on the way to visit Horiyoshi's tattoo museum in Yokohama. There we were, crazy tat-

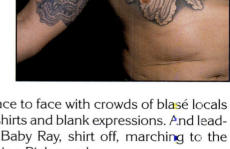

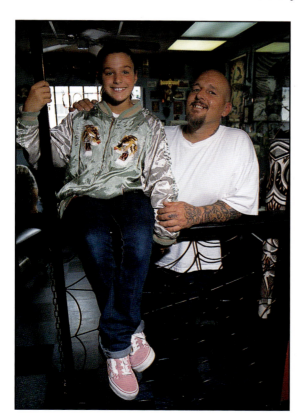

Baby Ray and his daughter Sarah.

tooed foreigners face to face with crowds of blasé locals with long-sleeved shirts and blank expressions. And leading the pack was Baby Ray, shirt off, marching to the train like Grant taking Richmond.

Baby Ray was born in 1958 on the Westside of Los Angeles, California. He grew up in Venice, Culver City, and Inglewood. Ray's relatives were artists: His grandfather was an illustrator and his dad a sign painter. When Ray was around ten, he hung out at a local biker bar. "I used to trip off the tattoos," says Ray. Later, when he saw his friend get tattooed, "I took a toothbrush, bent it, used an eight-track motor, a piece of guitar string and a ballpoint pen and began tattooing. I started on friends. I was intrigued. Never did I think of tattooing as a means to make money. That's one of the cool things about it—surprise, surprise!"

The majority of Ray's work is black and gray. "I'm a shader. I'm not immune to color, but if I use color, I keep it simple. All the old stuff is coming back, the *cholo* stuff. Guys fly from Japan to get a tattoo of a '63 Impala, a *cholo* clown and hood rats. One of the biggest joys and payment in tattoo is to watch. You do a piece, and they go to the mirror, look at themselves, do poses and feel so much better about themselves. It's a big responsibility to do a great tattoo. My living is based solely on customers being pleased with the piece—and the experience. Other than that, I'm nobody. Mr. Nobody."

Baby Ray is in a car club called the Beatniks made up primarily of tattooers like Jack Rudy, Brian Everett and some other friends. "I always liked cars, low riders, Harleys, that kind of stuff. I was really enthused with all of it. One time, some guy pulled up in a '49 Chevy, and it was like, wow! I feel very, very honored to be in this business. The people that live to tattoo are one big family. Tattoo isn't just my business, it's my life."

MR. GRUFF GUY

Even though he's got a gruff exterior, Baby Ray is one of the gentlest, most accommodating tattoo artists I've ever met. And it's reflected in his customers. I arrived at Spotlight on a Saturday morning, and, in a show of support for their artist, there was quite a crowd waiting for me. And, biggest surprise of all, Ray brought along his spunky little daughter, Sarah, who, with a little prodding from her dad, laid down a happy-face tattoo on one of the guys waiting to be photographed.

Ray drew the lines while Sarah pulled on the gloves. When it came to the actual tattooing, it was *zim, zam, zoom.* She must have completed that circle, dots for eyes and a smiley mouth in under two seconds!

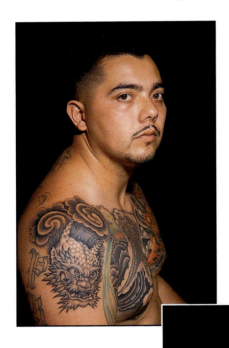

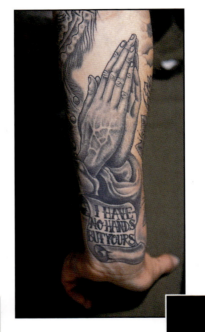

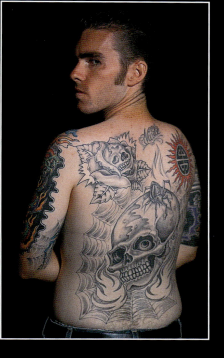
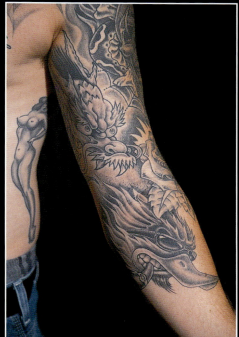
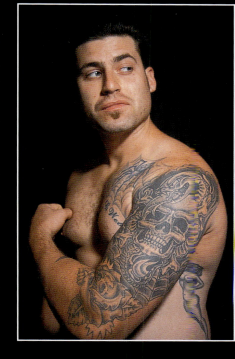
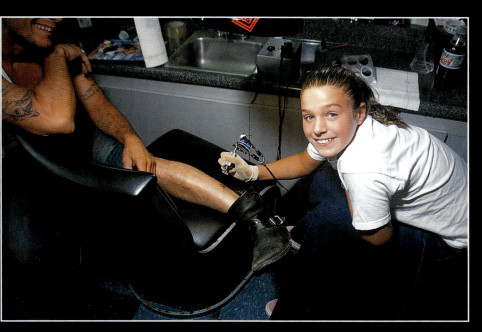
Sarah lays in a smiley face tattoo.
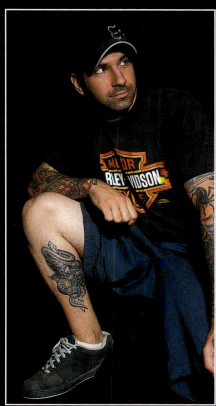

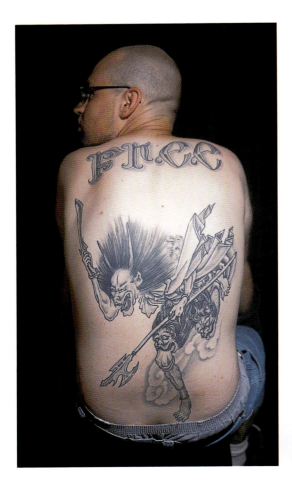

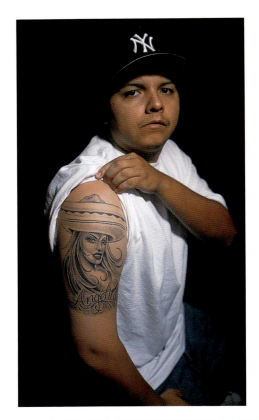

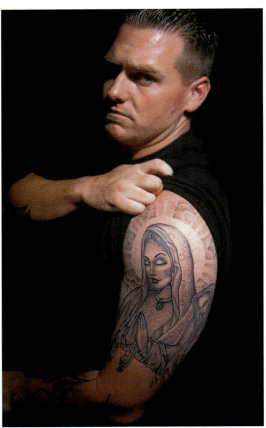

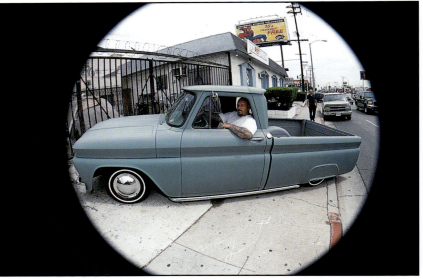

Ray and his rod.

"Slow down, slow down!" implored Ray. No use. It was over in a wink.

No worries. Ray was beaming from ear to ear. He couldn't have been prouder, although he may have some competition in the talented-daughter department. Bob Robert's daughter, Ava, is already working at the shop alongside her dad and brother, Charlie. When I visited Bob at his house, most of the talk was about Ava's artwork, and I got the complete tour of the watercolors, sketches and finger-painting that covered the walls.

Yep. Bob Roberts and Baby Ray. Two proud tattoo dads under the same roof.

ERIC MAASKE
CLASSIC TATTOO, FULLERTON

A visit to Eric Maaske's shop was a step back in time. From Maaske's greased-back hair and a cheek full of chaw to the '40s and '50s collectibles that decorate the walls, an afternoon with this master tattooist is truly an affirmation of the "classic" way of doing things. Under Maaske's scrutiny, every detail of the immaculate shop is designed to enhance the tattooing experience and make a visit to Fullerton unforgettable.

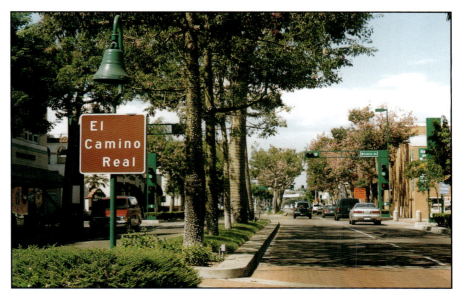

Midtown Fullerton.

Eric Maaske was born in Bellflower, California, in 1969. Eric's dad was covered in tattoos, which he got growing up in Chicago in the '50s. When Eric's dad got tattooed by Bob Shaw and Bud Graham at the Pike in Long Beach, California, Eric went along. He loved what he saw and, at the age of nine, tattooed some friends with a needle and thread. Eric built his first machine in '83 and tattooed his dad. At 14, he started tattooing on his own.

"I never expected to do it full time. I never thought I could make money doing tattoos. I just did it for fun on my friends."

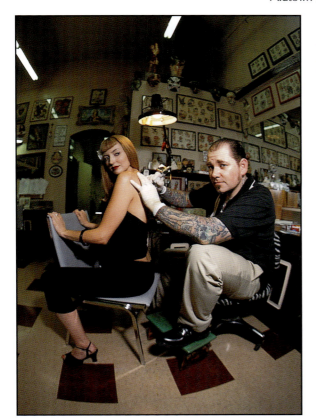

The elegant Mr. Maaske carries on the tradition.

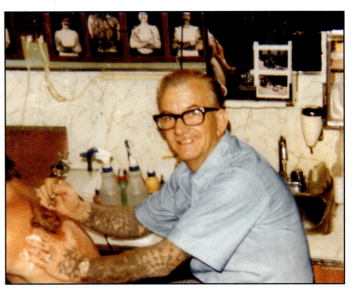

Bob Shaw tattooing, Long Beach, California, 1970s.
Photo courtesy of Tattoo Archive.

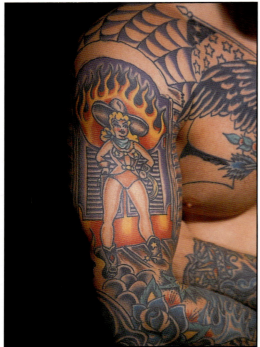

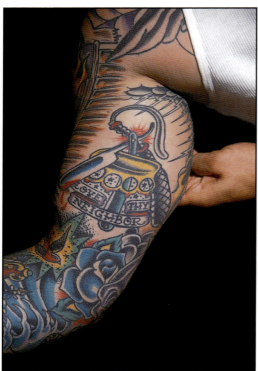

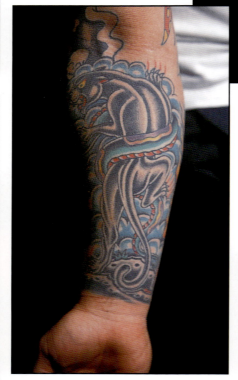

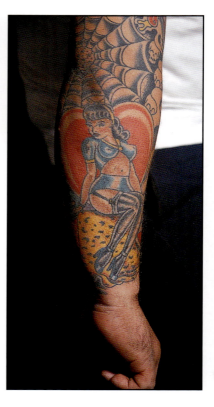

In 1990, Eric got hired in Newport Beach and a year later went to Classic Tattoo in Fullerton. He also worked for Dave Gibson in San Diego three days a week. "Aside from tattoos, Dave taught me a lot about painting. He taught me about ethics. When I was working with him, I was pretty new. I worked both shops seven days a week—four days in San Diego and three in Fullerton—for about a year." Eric ultimately bought Classic Tattoo in November of 2001.

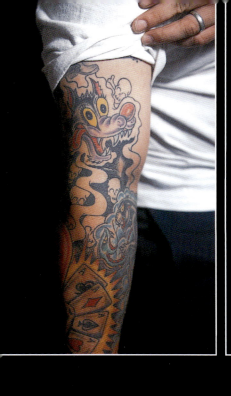
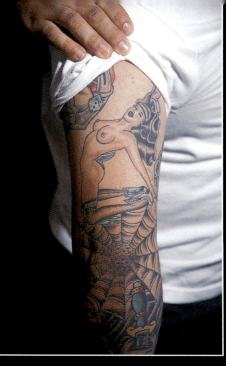
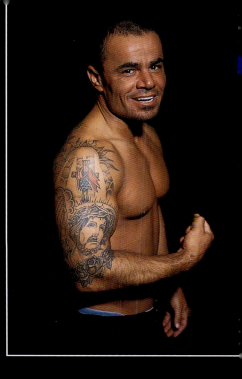
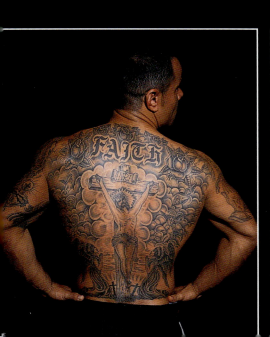
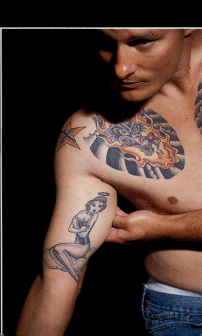
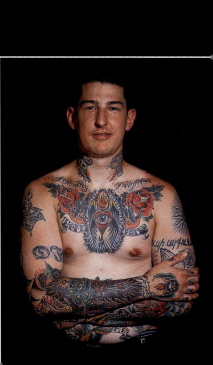

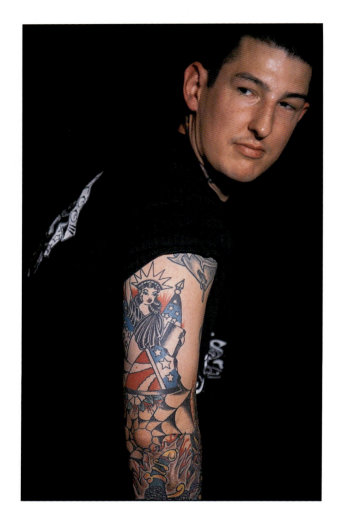
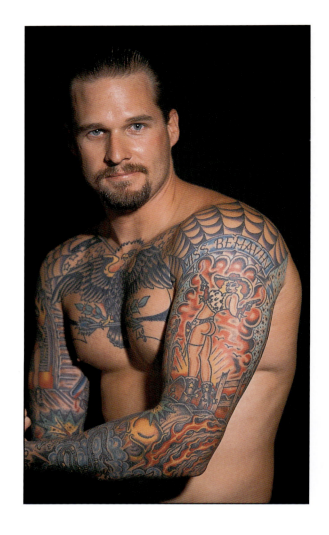
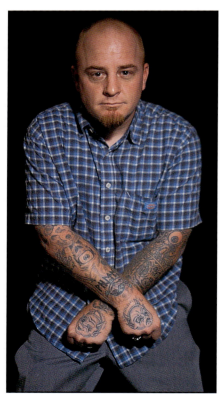
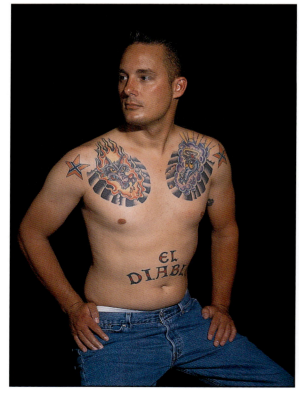

186

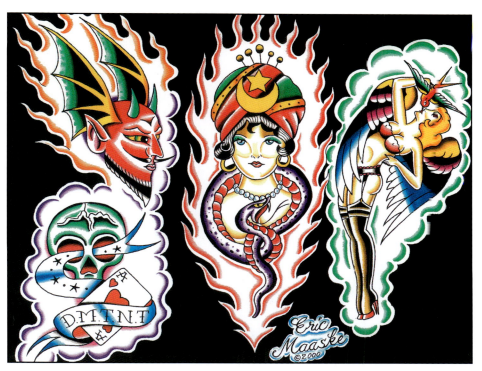

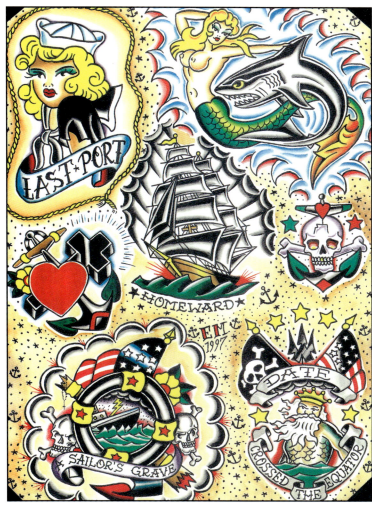

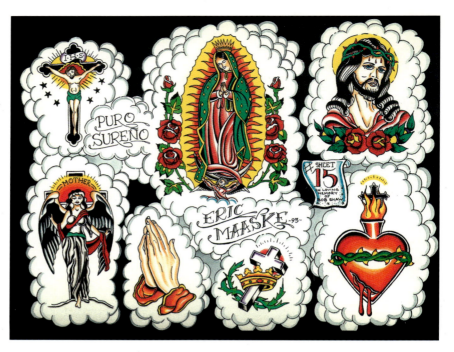

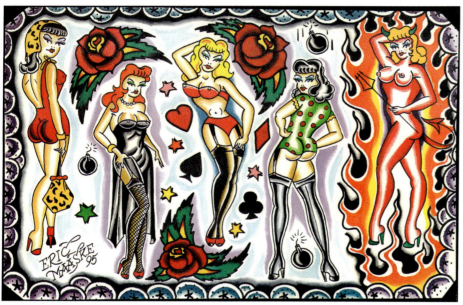

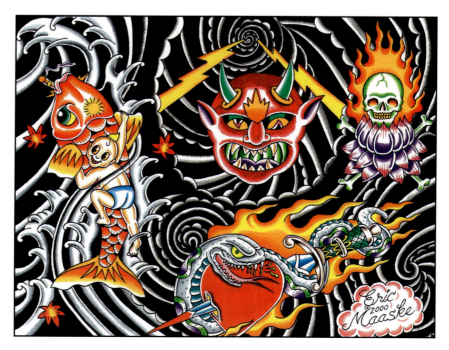

THE LAST STOP

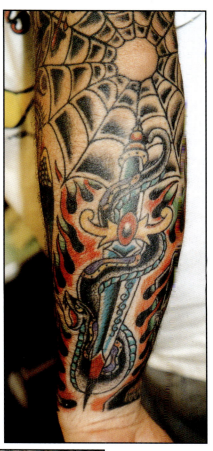

It was interesting to me that Fullerton was the last stop on my itinerary. Fullerton is clearly a town in transition. Beautifully laid out on the old El Camino Real, Fullerton harkens back to a time when main highways cut through the center of a town. As I drove down the tree-lined streets, many of the stores were closed or being revamped, in preparation, I guessed, for a resurgence of the old-time spirit. Many of the towns I visited are like this, returning to the look and feel of the glory days. And Eric Maaske fits right in. His high-ceilinged shop with the antique pinball machine and beauty-parlor chairs make a significant statement of the lasting way tattoo parlors are woven into the very fiber of the hometown community. Where once folks sat around the old cracker barrel, now it's the tattoo shop. And a great meeting place it is. While I was there, traveling artists dropped by just to say hello. Just to give a tip of the hat to the classic way of doing things in Old Town Fullerton. The way Eric Maaske does it.

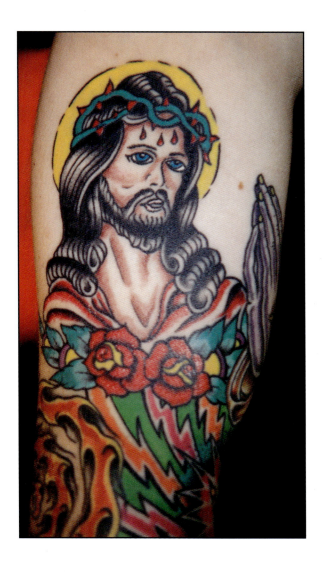

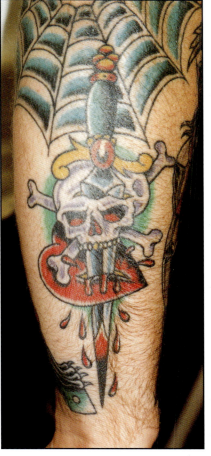

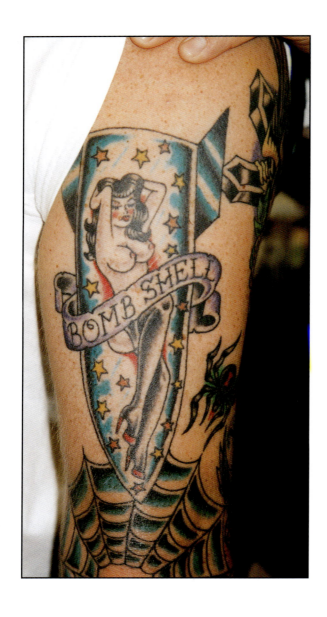

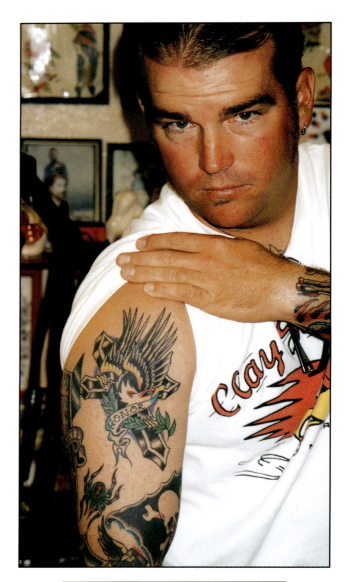

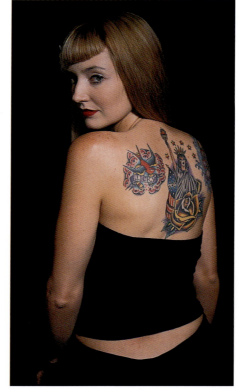

THE COMMEMORATIVE TATTOO

I decided to document each *Tattoo Road Trip* book with a tattoo. It started in Bend, Oregon, with *Tattoo Road Trip—The Pacific Northwest*. Gary Kosmala did a Haida-style beaver with a 1-shaped log in its mouth, to signify book one. Keone Nunes' Hawaiian design down my left leg will never let me forget the second in the series, *Two Weeks in Samoa*.

Now, for book number three.

Throughout this book are many amazing, old-guard, tried-and-true ink sinkers and trend-setting newcomers.

Who wouldn't want a tattoo by Jack, Greg, Mark, or Dave? The answer came to me, mid-adventure. Instead of a tattoo from an acknowledged legend, how about one from the *future* of tattooing? How about a tattoo that makes a statement about the future of the art form? And I couldn't think of anyone better than Jeremiah Barba. Still in his mid-20s, Jeremiah Barba has established himself as not only a top tattoo artist, but a significant creative force and, above all, a credit to himself, his family and the worldwide tattoo community.

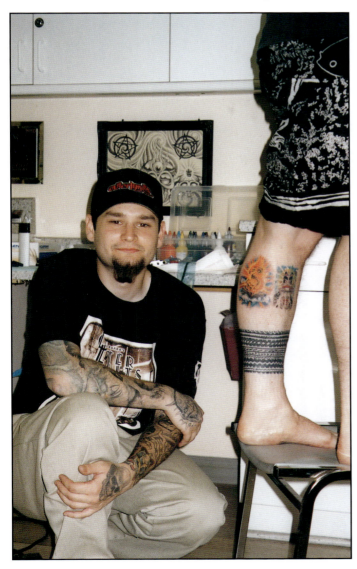

The artist.

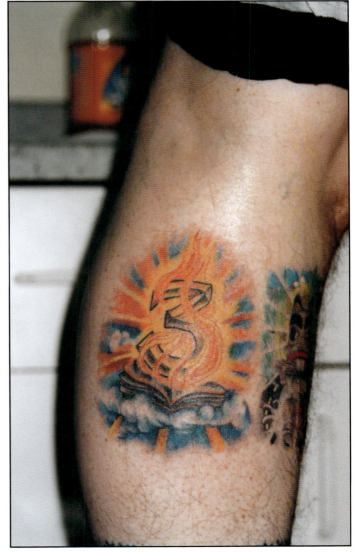

The tattoo.

EPILOGUE

I loved doing this book. Every time I entered a shop, I was welcomed like a long-lost brother. Some people had food, music blaring and, above all, a positive energy and a shop full of people. I also got a chance to spend some time with the artists. Some lay-back-and-gossip time. It was fun hearing all the stories, all the magical exploits that add the spice, the salt and pepper to the unfolding history of Southern California tattooing.

I let the story unfold naturally, from the mouths of the people who lived it. Tennessee Dave said it best: "Nowadays, I like the fact that everyone is more open." And that's the way it was. Instead of being excluded, I was a member, whether it was Jack Rudy or Mike Pike or Baby Ray. I felt a warm connection to these people. They know I love this business. They know I honor the traditions and immortalize the artists. That's such an important part of the tattoo life, apart from the travel and the creativity and the pirate lifestyle; it's the mem-bership in the extended family. Sure, this family is often dysfunctional, but the bloodlines are strong. The silent connections bring us together and unite us all. The scratch of the needle, the permanence of the ink, the roar of rock music, the smell of green soap the over-whelming ambiance. It's unforgettable.

This book captures a precious instant in time. A tick of the clock. The magic moment when new artists are emerging and others are becoming legends.

I deeply appreciate the many, many artists, shop staff and friends who have participated in this project. I espe-cially want to thank those who have always stood by me: my children, Jesse, Riley, Holly and Noah, my dear friend and soul mate Suzanne, C.W. Eldridge, Mr. Larry Flynt (who is a guiding light to us all) and the countless artists, collectors and historians who have both contrib-uted and inspired me on this wonderful adventure, this experience of a lifetime, this *Tattoo Road Trip*.

Bob Baxter
September 25, 2002
Pasadena, California

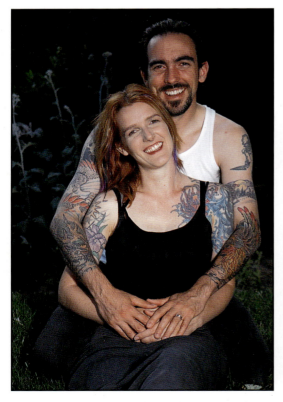

The author's daughter, Holly, and her husband, Conal. Tattoos by Rick Rockwood, Bob Roberts and Riley Baxter.

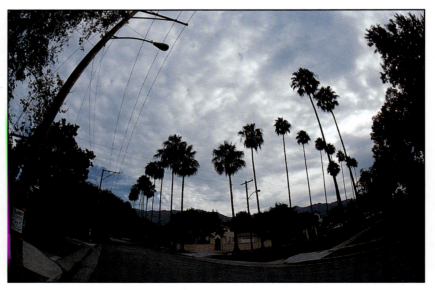